D0878176

THOMSON DELMAR LEARNING'S
NURSING REVIEW SERIES

Legal & Ethical Nursing

THOMSON DELMAR LEARNING'S
NURSING REVIEW SERIES

Legal & Ethical Nursing

Content taken from:
Delmar's Complete Review for NCLEX-RN®

By:
Donna F. Gauwitz, RN, MS
Nursing Consultant
Former Senior Teaching Specialist
School of Nursing
University of Minnesota Twin Cities
Minneapolis, Minnesota
Former Nursing Education Specialist
Mayo Clinic
Rochester, Minnesota

THOMSON
DELMAR LEARNING   Australia   Canada   Mexico   Singapore   Spain   United Kingdom   United States

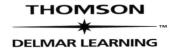

THOMSON

DELMAR LEARNING

™

Nursing Review Series: Legal & Ethical Nursing

by Donna F. Gauwitz

Vice President, Health Care Business Unit:
William Brottmiller

Director of Learning Solutions:
Matthew Kane

Acquisitions Editor:
Tamara Caruso

Product Manager:
Patricia Gaworecki

Editorial Assistant:
Jenn Waters

Marketing Director:
Jennifer McAvey

Marketing Channel Manager:
Michele McTighe

Marketing Coordinator:
Danielle Pacella

Technology Director:
Laurie Davis

Technology Project Manager:
Mary Colleen Liburdi
Patricia Allen

Production Director:
Carolyn Miller

Production Manager:
Barbara Bullock

Art Director:
Robert Plante
Jack Pendleton

Content Project Manager:
Dave Buddle
Stacey Lamodi
Jessica McNavich

Production Coordinator:
Mary Ellen Cox

Library of Congress Cataloging-in-Publication Data
ISBN 1-4018-1183-3

Notice to the Reader

Contents

Appendices

Contributors

Mary Mescher Benbenek, RN, MS, CPNP, CFNP
Teaching Specialist
School of Nursing
University of Minnesota
Twin Cities, Minnesota

Margaret Brogan, RN, BSN
Registered Nurse/Expert
Children's Memorial Hospital
Chicago, Illinois

Mary Lynn Burnett, RN, PhD
Assistant Professor of Nursing
Wichita State University
Wichita, Kansas

Corine K. Carlson, RN, MS
Assistant Professor
Department of Nursing
Luther College
Decorah, Iowa

Gretchen Reising Cornell, RN, PhD, CNE
Professor of Nursing
Utah Valley State College
Orem, Utah

Vera V. Cull, RN, DSN
Former Assistant Professor of Nursing
University of Alabama
Birmingham, Alabama

Laura DeHelian, RN, PhD, APRN, BC
Former Assistant Professor of Nursing
Cleveland State University
Cleveland, Ohio

Della J. Derscheid, RN, MS, CNS
Assistant Professor
Department of Nursing
Mayo Clinic
Mayo Clinic College of Nursing
Rochester, Minnesota

Ann Garey, MSN, APRN, BC, FNP
Carle Foundation Hospital
Urbana, Illinois

Beth Good, RN, MSN, BSN
Teaching Specialist
University of Minnesota
Minneapolis, Minnesota

Samantha Grover, RN, BSN, CNS
Psychiatric Mental Health Clinical Specialist
MeritCare Health System
Moorhead, Minnesota

Jeanne M. Harkness, RN, BA, MSN, BSN, AOCN
Clinical Practice Specialist
Jane Brattain Breast Center
Park Nicollet Clinic
St. Louis Park, Minnesota

Linda Irle, RN, MSN, APN, CNP
Coordinator, Maternal-Child Nursing
University of Illinois
Urbana, Illinois
Family Nurse Practitioner, Acute Care,
Carle Clinic,
Champaign, Illinois

Amy Jacobson, RN, BA
Staff Nurse
United Hospital
St. Paul, Minnesota

Nadine James, RN, PhD
Assistant Professor of Nursing
University of Southern Mississippi
Hattiesburg, Mississippi

Lisa Jensen, CS, MS, APRN
Salt Lake City VA Healthcare System
Salt Lake City, Utah

Ellen Joswiak, RN, MA
Assistant Professor of Nursing
Staff Nurse
Mayo Medical Center
Rochester, Minnesota

Betsy Ann Skrha Kennedy, RN, MS, CS, LCCE
Nursing Instructor
Rochester Community and Technical
    College
Rochester, Minnesota

Robin M. Lally, PhD, RN, BA, AOCN, CNS
Teaching Specialist; Office 6-155
School of Nursing
University of Minnesota
Twin Cities, Minnesota

Penny Leake, RN, PhD
Luther College
Decorah, Iowa

Barbara Mandleco, RN, PhD
Associate Professor & Undergraduate
    Program Coordinator
College of Nursing
Brigham Young University
Provo, Utah

Gerry Matsumura, RN, PhD, MSN, BSN
Former Associate Professor of Nursing
Brigham Young University
Provo, Utah

Alberta McCaleb, RN, DSN
Associate Professor
Chair, Undergraduate Studies
University of Alabama School of Nursing
University of Alabama at Birmingham
Birmingham, Alabama

JoAnn Mulready-Shick, RN, MS
Dean, Nursing and Allied Health
Roxbury Community College
Boston, Massachusetts

Patricia Murdoch, RN, MS
Nurse Practitioner
University of Illinois, Chicago
Urbana, Illinois

Jayme S. Nelson, RN, MS, ARNP-C
Adult Nurse Practitioner
Assistant Professor of Nursing
Luther College
Decorah, Iowa

Janice Nuuhiwa, MSN, CPON, APN/ CNS
Staff Development Specialist
Hematology/Oncology/Stem Cell
    Transplant Division
Children's Memorial Hospital
Chicago, Illinois

Kristen L. Osborn, MSN, CRNP
Pediatric Nurse Specialist
UAB School of Nursing
UAB Pediatric Hematology/Oncology
Birmingham, Alabama

Karen D. Peterson, RN, MSN, BSN, PNP
Pediatric Nurse Practitioner
Division of Endocrinology
Children's Memorial Hospital
Chicago, Illinois

Kristin Sandau, RN, PhD
Bethel University's Department of
    Nursing
United's John Nasseff Heart Hospital
Minneapolis, Minnesota

Elizabeth Sawyer, RN, BSN, CCRN
Registered Nurse
United Hospital
St. Paul, Minnesota

Lisa A. Seldomridge, RN, PhD
Associate Professor of Nursing
Salisbury University
Salisbury, Maryland

Janice L. Vincent, RN, DSN
University of Alabama School of Nursing
University of Alabama at Birmingham
Birmingham, Alabama

Margaret Vogel, RN, MSN, BSN
Nursing Instructor
Rochester Community & Technical
  College
Rochester, Minnesota

Mary Shannon Ward, RN, MSN
Children's Memorial Hospital
Chicago, Illinois

Preface

Congratulations on discovering the best new review series for the NCLEX-RN®! Thomson Delmar Learning's Nursing Review Series is designed to maximize your study in the core subject areas covered on the NCLEX-RN® examination. The series consists of 8 books:

Pharmacology

Medical-Surgical Nursing

Pediatric Nursing

Maternity and Women's Health Nursing

Gerontologic Nursing

Psychiatric Nursing

Legal and Ethical Nursing

Community Health Nursing

Each text has been developed expressly to meet your needs as you study and prepare for the all-important licensure examination. Taking this exam is a stressful event and constitutes a major career milestone. Passing the NCLEX is the key to your future ability to practice as a registered nurse.

Each text in the series is designed around the most current test plan for the NCLEX-RN® and provides a focused and complete content review in each subject area. Additionally, there are up to 400 review questions in each text: questions at the end of most every chapter and three 100 question review tests that support the chapter content. Each set of review questions is followed by answers and rationales for both the right and wrong answers. There is also a free PDA download of review questions available with the purchase of any of these review texts! It is this combination of content review and self assessment that provides a powerful learning experience for you as you prepare for you examination.

ORGANIZATION

Thomson Delmar Learning's unique Pharmacology review book provides you with an intensive review in this all important subject area. Drugs are grouped by classification and similarities to aid you in consolidating this pertinent but sometimes overwhelming information. Included in this text are:

- A section on herbal medicines, now being tested on the exam.
- Case studies that apply relevant drug content
- Prototypes for most drug classifications
- Mechanism of drug action
- Uses and adverse effects
- Nursing implications and discharge teaching
- Related drugs and their variance from the prototype

The review texts for Medical-Surgical Nursing, Pediatric Nursing, Maternity Nursing, Gerontological Nursing and Psychiatric Nursing follow a systematic approach that includes:

- The nursing process integrated with a body systems approach
- Introductory review of normal anatomy and physiology as well as basic theories and principles
- Review of pertinent disorders for each system including: general characteristics, pathophysiology/psychopathology
- Medical management
- Assessment data
- Nursing interventions and client education

Community Health Nursing and Legal and Ethical Nursing are unique review texts in the marketplace. They include aspects of community health nursing and legal/ethical subject matter that is covered on the NCLEX-RN® exam. Community Health topics covered are: case management, long-term care, home health care and hospice. Legal and ethical topics include: cultural diversity, leadership and management, ethical issues and legal issues for older adults.

FEATURES

All questions in each text in the series are compliant with the most current test plan from the National Council of State Boards of Nursing (NCSBN). All questions are followed by answers and rationales for both right and wrong choices. Included are many of the alternative format questions first introduced to the exam in 2003. An icon identifies these alternate types ●. The questions in each of these texts are written primarily at the application or analysis cognitive levels allowing you to further enhance critical thinking skills which are heavily weighted on the NCLEX.

In addition, with the purchase of any of these texts, a free PDA download is available to you. It provides you with up to an additional 225 questions with which you can practice your test taking skills.

Thomson Delmar Learning is committed to help you reach your fullest professional potential. Good luck on the NCLEX-RN® examination!

> To access your free PDA download for Thomson Delmar Learning's Nursing Review Series visit the online companion resource at **www.delmarhealthcare.com** Click on Online Companions then select the Nursing discipline.

Reviewers

Dr. Geri Beers, RN, EdD
Associate Professor of Nursing
Samford University
Birmingham, Alabama

Nancy D. Bingaman, RN, MS
Nursing Instructor
Maurine Church Coburn School of
    Nursing
Monterey Peninsula College
Monterey, California

Carol Boswell, EdD, RN
Associate Professor
College of Nursing
Texas Tech University Health Sciences
    Center
Odessa, Texas

Judy A. Bourrand, RN, MSN
Assistant Professor
Ida V. Moffett School of Nursing
Samford University
Birmingham, Alabama

Clara Willard Boyle, RN, BS, MS, EdD
Associate Professor
Salem State College
Salem, Massachusetts

Rebecca Gesler, MSN, RN
Assistant Professor
Spalding University
Louisville, Kentucky

Susan Hinck, PhD, RN, CS
Associate Professor
Department of Nursing
Missouri State University
Springfield, Missouri

Mary M. Hoke, PhD, APRN-BC
Academic Department Head
New Mexico State University
Las Cruces, New Mexico

Loretta J. Heuer, PhD, RN, FAAN
Associate Professor
College of Nursing
University of North Dakota
Grand Forks, North Dakota

Ann Putnam Johnson, EdD, RN
Professor of Nursing
Associate Dean, College of Applied
    Sciences
Western Carolina University
Cullowhee, North Carolina

Brenda P. Johnson, PhD, RN
Associate Professor, Dept. of Nursing
Southeast Missouri State
    University
Cape Girardeau, Missouri

Pat. S. Kupina, RN, MSN
Professor of Nursing
Joliet Junior College
Joliet, Illinois

Mary Lashley, RN, PhD, APRN, BC
Associate Professor
Department of Nursing
Towson University
Towson, Maryland

Melissa Lickteig, EdD, RN
Assistant Professor
School of Nursing
Georgia Southern University
Statesboro, Georgia

Caron Martin, MSN, RN
Associate Professor
School of Nursing and Health
  Professions
Northern Kentucky University
Highland Heights, Kentucky

**Darlene Mathis, MSN, RN, APRN, BC,
NP-C, CNE, CRNP**
Assistant Professor and Certified Nurse
  Educator
Samford University Ida V. Moffett School
  of Nursing
Family Nurse Practitioner
Birmingham Health Care
Birmingham, Alabama

Carol E. Meadows, MNSc, RNP, APN
Instructor
Eleanor Mann School of Nursing
University of Arkansas
Fayetteville, Arkansas

Margaret A. Miklancie, PhD, RN
Assistant Professor
College of Nursing & Health Science
George Mason University
Fairfax, Virginia

Frances D. Monahan, PhD, RN
Professor of Nursing
SUNY Rockland Community
  College
Consutant, Excelsior College

Deb Poling, MSN, APRN, BC, FNP, ANP
Assistant Professor
Regis University
Denver, Colorado
Case Manager
The Childrens Hospital
Denver, Colorado

Abby Selby, MNSc, RN
Faculty
Mental Health and Illness
Eleanor Mann School of Nursing
College of Education and Health Professions
University of Arkansas
Fayetteville, Arkansas
PRN educator
Mental Health Topics
Northwest Health System
Springdale, Arkansas

Sarah E. Shannon, PhD, RN
Associate Professor
Biobehavioral Nursing and Health Systems
Adjunct Associate Professor
Medical History and Ethics
University of Washington
Seattle, Washington

Susan Sienkiewicz, MA, RN
Professor
Community College of Rhode Island
Warwick, Rhode Island

Maria A. Smith, DSN, RN, CCRN
Professor
School of Nursing
Middle Tennessee State University
Murfreesboro, Tennessee

Ellen Stuart, MSN, RN
Professor
Mental Health Nursing
Grand Rapids Community College
Grand Rapids, Michigan

Karen Gahan Tarnow, RN, PhD
Faculty
School of Nursing
University of Kansas
Kansas City, Kansas

Janice Tazbir, RN, MS, CCRN
Associate Professor of Nursing
School of Nursing
Purdue University Calumet
Hammond, Indiana

Patricia C. Wagner, MSN, RNC
Clinical Assistant Professor
MCN Department, College of Nursing
University of South Alabama
Mobile, Alabama

Cultural Diversity

■ GUIDELINES FOR CULTURALLY SENSITIVE PRACTICE

A. Self examination – don't say an understanding has taken place if it hasn't
B. Use of Language – ask others how they wish to be addressed.
C. Body Language – find out what is appropriate, eye contact, touching, and distance
D. Don't Assume – find out who is involved and include them
E. Listen – what does the client know

■ KEY TERMS

1. Acculturation – the process of learning norms, beliefs, and behavioral expectations of a group. To acquire the majority group's culture.
2. Belief – basic assumptions or personal convictions that the individual believes are true.
3. Ethnocentrism – the belief that one's own culture is superior to all others.
4. Ethnicity – a cultural group's perception of themselves.
5. Generalizations – broad information about a culture.
6. Stereotype – fixed notion or conception of person or group with no allowance for individuality.
7. Cultural Competence – having the knowledge, understanding, and skills regarding a diverse culture that allow one to provide acceptable care.
8. Values – principles that have meaning and worth to an individual, family, group, or community.
9. Culture – values, beliefs, norms, and practices of a particular group that are learned, and shared and guide thinking, decision, and action in a patterned way.
10. Cultural Diversity – the differences in values, beliefs, norms, and practices between cultures.

NURSING ALERT

A culturally competent nurse must be ready to care for clients that may not be sensitive to the nurse's culture. We cannot judge others for not being culturally sensitive toward us.

11. Ancestry – refers to a person's nationality group, lineage, or the country in which the person or the person's parents or relatives were born before they came to the United States.
12. Socialization – process of being raised within a culture and acquiring the characteristics of the given group.
13. Emic – Person's way of describing an action or event, an inside view.
14. Etic – The interpretation of an event by someone who is not experiencing that event, an outside view.
15. Heritage Consistency – observance of the beliefs and practices of one's traditional cultural belief system.
16. Heritage Inconsistency – observance of the beliefs and practices of one's acculturated belief system.
17. Assimilation – to become absorbed into another culture and to adopt its characteristics, to develop a new cultural identity.

■ AFRICAN-AMERICAN
A. Communication
  1. Languages include English and Black English (a very expressive dialect spoken mainly in inner cities).
  2. Non-verbal communication
     a. May be affectionate – affection shown by hugging or touching but touching another's view may be viewed as offensive
     b. Direct eye contact may be viewed as rude
     c. Silence may indicate lack of trust for the caregiver
     d. Head-nodding does not necessarily mean agreement
     e. Non-verbal communication is very important
     f. May be viewed as intrusive to ask personal questions of someone that an individual has just met
B. Time Orientation
  1. Flexible time frame.
  2. Life issues may take priority over keeping appointments.
  3. Primarily present oriented
  4. Has a close personal space
C. Family Structure
  1. Extended, matriarchal, may include close friends in kin support system
  2. Large and extended families are important

CLIENT TEACHING CHECKLIST

When caring for culturally diverse clients, the client should understand:

- You are willing to personalize care that takes into account their culture.
- Questioning the client about their culture is necessary for you to understand the client's culture.
- They should notify you if something is not acceptable to them because of their culture.
- They should notify you of any herbal supplements and cultural practices used for illness prior to the hospitalization or visit.

NURSING ALERT

When caring for an African-American client, visiting restrictions, especially how many people can be in a room, may not fit within their extended family structure. You should attempt to utilize other rooms to accommodate visits.

    3. Father or eldest family member usually spokesperson.
    4. Elders are typically a source of wisdom and demand respect.
    5. Single-parent families may be female-headed households serving as both caretakers and breadwinner
D. Religion and Spirituality
    1. Religion mainly Protestant such as Baptist, however, some are followers of Islam and/or other faiths.
    2. Prayer and visits from minister common.
    3. Affiliation to church community is important.
    4. Faith and/or herbalism may be used in conjunction with biomedical therapy.
E. Dietary Practice
    1. Three meals daily including a large meal in late afternoon which is generally supper
    2. Prefer cooked foods such as pork that may not be eaten for religious reasons.
    3. Usual diet includes meat, fish, greens, rice, potatoes, corn, and yams
    4. Foods generally slow-cooked in added fat
    5. Some pregnant clients may participate in pica or the ingestion of food items such as starch used in laundry
F. Health and Illness Beliefs
    1. A belief that God, health, and illness are closely connected.

    2. A higher power extends to every facet of life including health.

    3. Illness can be classified as natural and unnatural.

        a. Natural illness has natural causes – caused by such things as exposure to cold air, rain, heat, impurities in the air, bad food or water such as arthritis pain.

        b. An unnatural illness is caused by evil influences on the person in the form of witch craft, hoodoo, voodoo or root work.

        c. Professional health care workers can work to treat or cure the natural illnesses.

        d. Generic or traditional healers work to treat unnatural illnesses.

    4. Proper diet, proper behavior, cleanliness, and exercise in fresh air maintain health.

G. Common Illnesses

    1. Hypertension

    2. Cardiovascular disease

    3. Stomach and esophageal cancer

    4. Lactose intolerance

    5. Sickle cell Anemia

H. Nursing Interventions

    1. Encourage the participation of the family

    2. Be aware that a folk healer or herbalist may be consulted before the client seeks treatment

    3. Explore with the client the meaning of their nonverbal behavior to validate their meaning

    4. Be flexible with the use of time and avoid rigidity in the scheduling of the client's care activities

    5. Verify the meaning and intent of the client's words

■ ASIAN-AMERICANS

A. Communication

    1. Languages include Chinese especially Mandarin, Japanese, Korean, Vietnamese, and English

    2. Non-verbal communication

        a. Quiet, polite, and tend not to disagree.

        b. Eye contact may be considered rude and is avoided with authority figures.

        c. Keeping a respectful distance is recommended.

        d. Silence is valued.

        e. Head nodding does not generally mean agreement.

        f. The head is considered sacred and should not be touched.

        g. Usually do not touch others, unacceptable to touch members of the opposite sex.

        h. An up-turned palm may be viewed as offensive

NURSING ALERT

W hen caring for Asian-American clients, it is important to rely on verbal answers for agreement instead of nodding or smiling.

B. Time Orientation
   1. Promptness important understanding the importance of keeping appointments.
   2. Oriented more to present.
C. Family Structure
   1. Extended families common, two or three generations often live in the same household.
   2. A clan is another form of family structure. A clan is a recognized grouping of families with the same last name and line of ancestors.
   3. Family unit is very structured and hierarchical.
   4. Men have power and authority and women are obedient but women have strong influence in the home.
   5. Elder very respected and honored.
   6. Education highly valued.
D. Religion and Spirituality
   1. Religions include Buddhism, Islam, Catholicism, Protestant, and Taoism.
   2. Buddhists practice act of Dana (generosity), believed to return to them in the future as karma.
   3. Catholics pray, recite the rosary and may consult the chaplain.
   4. Some practice ancestor veneration, believing the deceased go to a place near the living and are able to help or hinder the living relatives.
   5. May have an altar for ancestor worship.
   6. Some Chinese use herbalists and acupuncturists in conjunction with western medicine
   7. May believe in reincarnation.
E. Dietary Practice
   1. Usually eat three meals a day with many preferring to use chopsticks.
   2. Diet usually low in fat, animal protein, cholesterol and sugar.
   3. Fish, soybeans, vegetables, rice, noodles, and soy sauce
   4. Generally prefer tea, coffee, and water because many Asians are lactose intolerant.
   5. For Chinese, food is viewed as important in maintaining balance of yin (cold) and yang (hot) in the body. Food used to treat illness and disease.
   6. Yin foods which have a positive energy force includes fruits, vegetables, and cold liquids.
   7. Yang foods which have a negative energy force include meat, eggs, hot soup and liquids, oily and fried foods.

NURSING ALERT

C upping is often performed to the back and is apparent by round bruises. You should document these finding in the skin assessment.

F. Health and Illness Belief.
   1. Health is a state of physical and spiritual harmony with nature.
   2. Health is also maintaining balance between yin and yang influences, not only in the body but also in the environment.
   3. Most physical illnesses caused by imbalance of yin and yang
   4. Chronic illness may be attributed to karma and may result from bad behavior in this life or in past life
   5. Herbal remedies such as ginseng commonly used for anemia, colic, depression, or indigestion.
   6. Preventing illness and promoting health, one should eat a diet balanced with yin and yang foods.
   7. Practices such as pinching, coining (rubbing a coin over the skin causing a mark), cupping (applying a glass over the skin, suction created, causes the skin to rise up and turn blue) are believed to let the unhealthy air currents out of the body.
   8. A body that is healthy may be viewed as a gift from the ancestors
G. Common Illnesses
   1. Hypertension
   2. Lactose intolerance
   3. Stomach and liver cancer
H. Nursing Interventions
   1. Avoid direct eye contact and gesturing with the hands
   2. Avoid excessive touching and before touching the client's head explain why it is necessary to do so
   3. Be aware that the client may consult a traditional healer before a client consults modern medicine
   4. Explore with client their responses to questions
   5. Be flexible with the use of time and avoid extreme rigidity when scheduling cares

■ HISPANIC AMERICANS

A. Communication
   1. Languages include Spanish or Portuguese with may dialects present
   2. Direct confrontation is considered disrespectful
   3. Impolite to have an expression of negative feelings
   4. Confidentiality is important
   5. Very tactile and a hand shake or embrace is often used

NURSING ALERT

nvolving family in the care of the Hispanic-American client and having them assist in care such as personal hygiene may help the family deal with an illness.

6. Politeness and modesty are valued
7. Non-verbal communication.
   a. Gestures are often used
   b. Eye contact avoided typically with authority figures and indicates respect and attentiveness
   c. Touch especially by strangers is unappreciated.
   d. Silence may indicate lack of agreement and tend to be verbally expressive
   e. Emotions or pain is expressed through dramatic body gestures or facial expressions
B. Time Orientation
   1. Present oriented
   2. Flexible time frame
   3. Comfortable with a closeness to other individuals
C. Family Structure
   1. Generally patriarchal with males making the decisions and money and females managing the household.
   2. Families are typically large and include extended relatives.
   3. Loyalty and obligation to family important.
   4. The elderly are respected and children are expected to obey their parents
   5. Taking care of elder parents is seen as a privilege not an obligation
D. Religion and Spirituality
   1. Roman Catholic predominant religion
   2. A worldview that one must accept what God gives. A common belief that whatever happens is God's will.
   3. Religious ceremonies important such as baptism and marriage.
   4. Prayers common, statues, crosses, and candles evident in many homes
   5. Health may result from a state of balance between "hot" and "cold" forces or "wet" and "dry forces"
   6. Illness may be viewed as a punishment for their sins
E. Dietary Practices
   1. The main meal is usually at noon.
   2. Rice, beans, corn, and chilies are staple foods.
   3. Fried and spicy foods are consumed
F. Health and Illness Beliefs
   1. In time of illness, individuals may utilize biomedical and folk health systems

---

DELEGATION TIP

When delegating care of the culturally diverse client, you must include information about the client's practices to assist in providing culturally competent care from all members of the health care team.

---

2. Self-medication and use of "curandera" (folk healer) are common
3. Other traditional healers include Yerberos (herbalists) and sobadores (masseuses)
4. Traditional diseases include:
   a. Empacho—stomach upset caused by eating wrong foods at wrong time of day or eating undercooked foods.
   b. Caida de mollera—sunken fontanel caused by pulling baby away from breast or bottle too quickly, carrying the baby incorrectly or from the baby falling.
   c. Susto—fright sickness caused by a traumatic or frightening experience.
   d. Mal ojo—evil eye caused by a person with a "strong eye' that touches a child while. admiring them.
   e. Mal puesto—when someone uses witchcraft to put a bad disease in a person.
5. Many individuals will not discuss their folk healing remedies with the professional health care provider out of respect.
G. Common Illnesses
   1. Parasite infestation
   2. Lactose intolerance
   3. Diabetes
H. Nursing Interventions
   1. Display a non-judgemental attitude regarding the folk healing therapies and obtain as much information regarding herbs and/or supplements used
   2. Offer to call a priest when the client is ill
   3. Maintain privacy and confidentiality
   4. Communication is generally through the head of the family
   5. Use a gesture of touch when examining a child
   6. Be flexible when scheduling care and avoid extreme rigidity

■ NATIVE AMERICANS

A. Communication—depends on tribal group and bands such as Navajos, Lakota, Sioux and Ojibwa
   1. Languages
      a. There are over 150 spoken Native American languages, although most speak English as well.

NURSING ALERT

I t may be difficult for the American Indian to make and keep appointments because of their casual view of time. You should realize this behavior is not non-compliance but a cultural norm.

     b. Many of the languages involve a tonal speech in which the pitch is of great importance.

     c. Frequently use metaphors or anecdotes when speaking and many times the Indian language does not have an equivalent single English word for translation.

     d. Typical speech pattern is slow with low tone of voice.

  2. Non-verbal communication.

     a. Maintain little eye contact – eye contact is considered a sign of disrespect.

     b. Silence is acceptable, viewed as positive, and a sign of respect for the speaker

     c. It is very important to remain attentive during conversations and it is considered rude to indicate the person was not heard or to interrupt the speaker.

     d. Note taking during conversations or interviews is generally not acceptable.

     e. Lightly touching the hand when meeting or greeting a person is acceptable

     f. Body language is an important mode of communication

B. Time Orientation

  1. Present-time oriented.

  2. Time may be viewed as being on a continuum, with no beginning and no end.

C. Family Structure

  1. Extremely family oriented – the term "family" typically involves all members of the extended family such as first cousins being treated as brothers or sisters

  2. Usually a male family member with the greatest amount of prestige will rise as "leader" for the extended family and provide direction.

  3. Elders are highly respected and pass many of the traditions down to younger members.

  4. Children are taught to respect traditions and to honor wisdom.

  5. Mother is typically responsible for domestic duties.

  6. Common for large extended family to visit a patient in the hospital.

  7. Personal space is very important with space having no boundaries

  8. Massage is used to promote bonding between a mother and the infant

  9. Community social organizations are viewed as important

D. Religion and Spirituality
  1. Religious affiliation and practices are an individual decision.
  2. Both traditional and a variety of Christian religions are practiced.
  3. Sacred myths and legends are often valued
  4. Religion and practices in healing go together
E. Dietary Practice
  1. Influenced by tribal beliefs, geographical area, and availability.
  2. Traditional diets in the past consisted of low fat, such as fruits, berries, roots, fish, game and wild greens.
  3. The traditional diet has transformed due to the scarcity of these foods in federally defined Indian geographical regions.
  4. Modern, processed foods, high in fat and sugar more common now.
  5. Lactose intolerance common because many people do not drink milk.
  6. Alcohol abuse is a concern because Native Americans exhibit high risk behaviours related to alcohol abuse.
  7. Corn is an important staple in the diet.
F. Health and Illness Beliefs
  1. Health is believed to reflect harmony with the surrounding environment and family.
  2. Traditional health beliefs focus on wellness and wholeness.
  3. Traditional remedies may include an act of purification such as immersion in water, sweat lodges, herbal medicines, and special rituals.
  4. Herbs and roots are considered agents of nature or spiritual helpers and are used medicinally.
  5. Medicine man may be consulted and is considered an important part of treatment.
  6. Symbolic or sacred items such as feathers, stones, arrowheads, corn pollen maybe used for healing and blessing.
  7. Both traditional and western medicine may be utilized.
  8. It is forbidden to touch a dead body
G. Common Illnesses
  1. Cardiovascular disease
  2. Diabetes
  3. Arthritis
  4. Glaucoma
  5. Tuberculosis
H. Nursing Interventions
  1. Encourage the participation of family members
  2. Encourage the client to bring personal items into the hospital to personalize the space
  3. Explore messages for clarification
  4. Understand that although eye contact may be absent that the client is attentive

■ ARAB-MIDDLE EAST AMERICANS

A. Communication
   1. Languages include Arabic (variations exist in dialects) and English is also widely spoken.
   2. Non-verbal communication.
      a. Warm, shy, and modest.
      b. When one feels accepted and trusted, they tend to be more expressive.
      c. Prefer closeness in space and with the same sex.
      d. Typically very polite and may respond in ways to make others happy.
      e. When men greet, hugging and kissing is common.
B. Time Orientation
   1. Past and present oriented.
   2. Typically "on time" for business issues, more casual and spontaneous for informal gatherings.
C. Family Structure
   1. The family is the strongest social unit in Arab culture.
   2. Typically the Arab family is patrilineal consisting of the father's brother's families, grandparents on the father's side, and children.
   3. At times of crises, family members show support financially and through their presence.
   4. The concept of honor and shame strongly influence the family.
   5. Mothers, sisters, daughters, grandmothers provide the caring functions.
   6. Father, eldest son or uncle usually family spokesperson.
   7. Elders are respected.
   8. Children are sacred and expected to be obedient. More strict with girls than boys.
D. Religion and Spirituality
   1. Majority of Arabs immigrating to the United States are Muslims.
   2. Majority of Arabs in Middle East are Muslims.
   3. Muslim (followers of Islam) greatly affects the lives of Arabs.
   4. The Islamic holy book is the Quran.
   5. Islam is based on five religious duties referred to as pillars:
      a. Profession of faith.
      b. Prayer five times daily facing Mecca.
      c. Fasting during Ramadan—Muslims do not eat, drink or smoke from sunrise to sunset. Meals are served at night.
      d. Almsgiving (usually 2.5% of a person's total net worth).
      e. Pilgrimage to the Holy City of Mecca.
E. Dietary Practice
   1. A healthy, hearty diet is important.
   2. Fruits, vegetables and breads are common.
   3. Meats usually consist of chicken and lamb served with rice or soup.

NURSING ALERT

When caring for a Muslim client, you should help the client identify which direction is facing Mecca and provide washcloths and towels to help them cleanse before praying.

4. At home the meal is served with people typically sitting on the floor.
5. The meal is often eaten quickly and in silence.
6. Under Islamic law, the consumption of alcohol and improperly slaughtered meat is forbidden.

F. Health and Illness Beliefs
   1. The strong religious foundation of Arab is important to understand as this guides their health and illness belief system.
   2. A belief that God or prophet Muhammed is omnipotent and cause for all health and illness.
   3. If one loses faith in God, then illness may befall that person.
   4. A person is healthy if they are in harmony with God.
   5. Family members and close friends accompany clients to the hospital and expect to participate in care or take an overseeing role.
   6. Arab sometimes have difficulty questioning medical authorities and being actively involved in medical decision making and often expect the physician to make medical decisions
   7. Highly technical, invasive therapies are seen as superior to non-invasive treatments.
   8. Immediate pain relief is expected and may be persistently requested.
   9. The belief in conserving energy for recovery is in conflict with therapies that require exertion.
   10. Home remedies include sweating rituals, religious verses, prayers, a well-balanced diet.
   11. Folk remedies include herbs, ointments, foods, enemas.

G. Common Illnesses
   1. Hypertension
   2. Cancer

H. Nursing Interventions
   1. Be aware that the client will be persistent in the request for pain medication
   2. Be aware that the client may resort to home remedies before seeking medical treatment
   3. Be supportive of client's religious preferences
   4. Encourage the client to be a participant in the health care

■ EUROPEAN AMERICANS

A. Communication
  1. Language
   Speak their national dialects

   English is widely spoken as a second language
  2. Non-verbal communication.
     a. Avoid close physical contact
     b. Direct eye contact used and indicates trustworthiness
     c. Handshake for greeting appreciated and develops trust.
     d. Nodding is a gesture of approval.
     e. Silence may be used for either a sign of respect or disdain depending on the circumstances
B. Time Orientation
  1. Most future oriented looking to the future
C. Family Structure
  1. Family oriented, extended family members often live together, relying on each other for financial and emotional support, child care, and household tasks.
  2. The father tends to have the greatest influence and makes decisions
  3. Children primarily are cared for by mother or grandmother.
  4. Education, family and cultural activities are highly valued.
  5. The individual is typically hard working, self reliant, and independent.
  6. Elders are highly respected.
D. Religion and Spirituality
  1. Mainly Judeo-Christian
E. Dietary Practice
  1. Diet is high in carbohydrates with bread being a staple
  2. High intake of red meat
F. Health and Illness Beliefs
  1. Views health as the absence of disease
  2. May use home remedies before consulting modern medicine
  3. May view illness as a negative force in their life and a result of their sins
  4. May be stoic when presenting with physical complaints
G. Common Illnesses
  1. Cardiovascular disease
  2. Diabetes
  3. Thalassemia
  4. Breast cancer
H. Nursing Interventions
  1. Pay particular attention to the client's body language
  2. Offer support to the client while attempting to decrease their negative view of illness
  3. Encourage client to consult modern medicine

NURSING ALERT

The European-American client may have difficulties following therapeutic diets because of the high carbohydrate, fat, and salt content in their diet. You should attempt to work with the client to find foods that are both acceptable for the client and conducive to their therapeutic diet.

REVIEW QUESTIONS

1. The outpatient care nurse is discussing postoperative dismissal teaching with an Asian-American client. During the discussion, the client looks at the floor, smiles at times, and nods his head. The nurse interprets this nonverbal behavior as

    1. an acceptance of the dismissal instructions.
    2. an understanding of the material taught.
    3. a reflection of cultural values.
    4. an ability to follow through with instructions.

2. The nurse in the emergency room is evaluating a head laceration on an 8-year-old Asian-American client. Prior to the physical assessment, the nurse should

    1. ask the parents to step out of the room.
    2. ask permission to examine the head.
    3. touch the child gently, explaining the procedure.
    4. discuss the dismissal care of a laceration.

3. The admission nurse is gathering family information on an Asian-American client. The client mentions the term "clan." The nurse understands this term to mean

    1. a group of friends and relatives that accompanied the client.
    2. the client's spouse.
    3. a sacred symbol the client wishes to keep nearby at all times.
    4. a recognized group of families with the same last name and line of ancestors.

4. The nursing instructor is describing the Chinese-American philosophy of *yin* and *yang* to a group of nursing students. The instructor describes how foods are classified using this belief system. Which of the following statements should the nursing instructor include that correctly describes the *yin* and *yang* food correlation?

1. *Yin* foods are hot
2. *Yin* and *yang* deals with energy, not food
3. *Yang* foods are cold
4. Cold foods are consumed when a hot illness is present

5. The nurse in the urgent care center is assessing an Asian-American adolescent with complaints of a sore throat. When auscultating lung sounds, the nurse notices round bluish marks along each side of the client's back. The nurse reports this as which of the following?

1. A potential skin infection
2. A sign of abuse
3. The practice of cupping
4. An allergy to a medication

6. During a care conference involving the nurse, physician, social worker, Asian-American client, and Asian-American family members, some suggestions for further care are being discussed. The client is sitting in a chair at the edge of the room. The client looks only at the family and does not speak during the conference. The nurse assesses the client's behavior as

[ ] 1. a withdrawal from the situation.
[ ] 2. a sign of denial regarding the condition.
[ ] 3. a lack of understanding of the discussion.
[ ] 4. a sign of respect for members of the health care team.

7. The nurse is reviewing follow-up instructions with an African-American client. The nurse notices that the client has missed two follow-up appointments in the last week. The client states "something else came up." The nurse interprets this as

1. a lack of understanding of the follow-up routine.
2. uncertainty of the willingness of the client to pursue further care.
3. a sense of noncommitment toward the plan of care.
4. a cultural value of a flexible time frame.

8. An African-American client with hypertension is attending a class on ways to take control of hypertension. The nurse explains dietary measures that can be used to help control blood pressure. Which of the following indicates the client has understood the material presented?

1. "I love fried chicken, but will choose broiled skinless chicken as my entrée."
2. "It is okay to use table salt, just not too much."

3. "I can still drink wine or beer with my dinner; these fluids don't interfere with blood pressure."

4. "I've never been a big vegetable eater; I don't suppose I need to start now."

9. An older adult African-American client has just received a diagnosis of prostate cancer. During a discussion with the family and nurse, the client states, "This is all in God's hands now; there's not much more I can do." The nurse interprets this statement as the client

   1. accepts the diagnosis.

   2. gives up on a possible cure.

   3. expresses feelings of loss of control.

   4. expresses a cultural belief in the connectedness of God, health, and illness.

10. The nurse is caring for an African-American client who recently had a hysterectomy. The client requests certain herbs from the dietician to be included with meals. When the meals arrive, the client and the faith healer perform a ritual over the herbs. The nurse assesses this as

    1. an unacceptable event and reports it to the charge nurse.

    2. a common practice to combine herbs, faith healing, and Western medicine.

    3. a way for the client to think she has control.

    4. a way for the client to individualize her own care.

11. The nurse in the diagnostic imaging center is preparing an African-American client with a history of headaches for a CT scan. Which of the following questions should the nurse avoid asking during the initial assessment?

    1. "Do you experience vision changes?"

    2. "Do you experience shortness of breath?"

    3. "Do you have a close relationship with your family?"

    4. "Do you typically experience headaches daily?"

12. The nurse is involved in discharge planning for an older Hispanic-American client with a terminal illness. The nurse offers services, such as Meals on Wheels, nursing care, and hospice. The client's family insists on providing all the care. The nurse identifies this situation as

    1. an unrealistic expectation for members of the family.

    2. an inability to accept other forms of help.

    3. a common practice, since it is often seen as a privilege when family members care for older adults.

    4. a way for family to stay in control of the older adult client.

13. A home health nurse is visiting a Hispanic-American client who does not speak English. A translator is not available at the time of the visit. The best approach for the nurse to overcome the language barrier is to

   1. discuss one issue at a time.

   2. write the medical terms down.

   3. offer to return at a different time.

   4. use simple words, gestures, and pictures.

14. A Hispanic-American client arrived at the emergency room complaining of severe stomach pains and cramps. Upon evaluation, the client described to the nurse a home remedy that included massage, prayer, rubbing, and gently pinching the spine. The nurse interpreted this behavior as

   1. an extreme attempt to avoid visiting a physician.

   2. an example of traditional folk remedies accepted by the Hispanic-American culture.

   3. a denial of the seriousness of the medical condition.

   4. an alternative approach with no scientific basis.

15. The nurse informs another nurse that which of the following statements best describes American Indians' beliefs about health?

   1. "The earth gives food, shelter, and medicine to humankind, and all things of the earth belong to human beings and nature."

   2. "Health is believed to reflect internal harmony."

   3. "Traditional health beliefs focus on illness and achieving health through nature."

   4. "The human body is viewed as several parts working together to attain health."

16. The nurse is explaining preoperative information to an American Indian client. The nurse observes the client to be quiet, looking at the picture on the wall, and not readily responding to the nurse's questions. This behavior would indicate the client

   1. is not accepting the information.

   2. has a hearing impairment.

   3. is listening to the nurse.

   4. is focusing on the environment.

17. The nurse admitting an American Indian client is working on the admission forms. The nurse has asked the client to speak louder and to repeat several comments. The client gets frustrated and won't continue the interview. Which of the following best describes this interaction?

1. The nurse was unaware of acceptable forms of communication with Indian clients

2. The client was feeling rushed during the interview process

3. The nurse was seeking clarification during the interview

4. The client was uncertain about the interview process

18. A nurse teaching a class on the characteristics of an Arab-American family unit uses the term patrilineal. The nurse should include which of the following statements to best describe patrilineal?

    1. A concept of honor or shame in the family

    2. A philosophy of time orientation specific to the Arab culture

    3. A special bond evident in most Arab families

    4. A family group consisting of family members on the father's side

19. A nurse is reviewing a diet with an Arab-American client. The nurse understands which of the following foods are typical in the Arab diet? Select all that apply:

    [ ] 1. Fried foods

    [ ] 2. Rice

    [ ] 3. Canned processed foods

    [ ] 4. Soup

    [ ] 5. Chicken

    [ ] 6. Lamb

20. The nurse is teaching a class on the cultural aspects of the Arab-American client. Which of the following should the nurse include in this class?

    1. Friends are the strongest social unit in the Arab-American culture

    2. The majority of Arabs immigrating to the United States are Muslims

    3. Following Islam has no effect on the lifestyles of Arab Americans

    4. Mealtime is a social time of long duration

21. An Arab-American client is referred for continuing care related to dizziness and vision changes. The nurse understands that an Arab-American client would prefer which of the following therapies as a treatment of the condition?

    1. Continued monitoring of the clinical manifestations

    2. CT scan of the head

    3. Blood work to check electrolytes

    4. Vision screening

22. A nurse caring for an Arab-American client is assessing the client's pain following angiography. The client is lying in bed, eyes tightly closed, and

continually asks for more pain medication. The client states, "I asked for pain medication right away and I need it now!" Which of the following nursing actions would be most appropriate at this time?

1. Check to see when the pain medication was last given
2. Explain to the client that the nurse was not aware of the discomfort
3. Try to obtain more information regarding the pain
4. Inform the client that the pain medication will be administered after assisting another client

23. Which of the following should the nurse include in a class on the health belief system associated with clients of the Russian-American culture?

1. A belief that man has little control over nature
2. A belief that God's will is the only will
3. A belief that nature, environment, and man are directly linked to health and wellness
4. A belief that eating right will maintain health

24. A nurse educator is working with staff on cultural diversity issues related to nonverbal communication. The educator explains to another nurse that appropriate nonverbal communication in the Russian-American culture includes which of the following?

1. Nodding is a gesture of approval
2. Handshakes are avoided
3. Direct eye contact is avoided
4. Touch is considered an invasion of privacy

25. A care conference is scheduled to discuss the prognosis of a terminally ill Russian-American client. The family members insist the client not be told the diagnosis. The nurse interprets this behavior as

1. unacceptable because every client has a right to personal medical information.
2. an ethical violation on the part of the family.
3. a typical response in Russian-American cultural tradition dealing with terminal illness.
4. a dishonest way of communicating.

ANSWERS AND RATIONALES

1. 3. In the Asian-American culture, eye contact is avoided with authority figures. Head nodding does not necessarily reflect agreement. Direct eye contact is frequently viewed as rude. The Asian-American culture typically avoids confrontation. The word "no" is avoided because it would show disrespect.

2. 2. In the Asian-American culture, the head is considered sacred. Touching the head is seen as disrespectful. Permission must be sought to touch the client. The parents should remain with the child to offer comfort and support.

3. 4. In the Asian-American culture, a clan is a family structure that includes a group of individuals considered ancestors and who have the same last name.

4. 4. In the Chinese-American culture, foods are classified as hot or cold and are transformed into *yin* and *yang* energy when metabolized by the body. *Yin* and *yang* represent a balance between positive and negative forces. *Yin* foods are cold and *yang* foods are hot. Cold foods are eaten when a hot illness is present. Hot foods are eaten when a cold illness is present.

5. 3. In the Asian-American culture, cupping involves applying a glass over the skin to create a suction that causes the skin to swell and turn bluish. This practice is believed to let the unhealthy air currents out of the body. If an allergy to a medication existed, the rash typically would be located in more areas than just the back. Further investigation and discussion would be necessary before abuse could be suspected.

6. 4. The Asian-American culture is typically viewed as quiet, polite, avoiding direct eye contact. Silence is valued and maintaining a distance is respected. Nonverbal communication is very important.

7. 4. A characteristic of African-American culture is the concept of time as flexible. The present takes precedent over the future. Members of the cultural group avoid rigidly scheduled appointments.

8. 1. In the African-American culture, clients typically enjoy fried, fatty foods. They slow-cook foods in added fat. The client has made an appropriate alteration to this food choice by choosing broiled skinless chicken over fried chicken. Salt and alcohol should be avoided. Encouraging fresh fruits and vegetables is also appropriate.

9. 4. In the African-American culture, there is a strong belief in God. They view God, health, and illness as being interconnected.

10. 2. It is common in the African-American culture to combine Western medicine with other traditions. An herbalist or folk healer may be consulted before an individual seeks traditional medicine. Certainly the patient has a right to request herbs and a faith healer. This activity would not warrant the charge nurse being notified.

11. 3. In the African-American culture, it is considered intrusive to ask personal questions during the initial assessment. Asking a client about having vision changes, shortness of breath, or headaches is physiologically based; these questions take priority during the admission process.

12. 3. In the Hispanic-American culture, older adults are respected and honored. Extended families typically live together and provide care as

necessary. This is seen as a privilege, not an obligation. Family members encourage involvement of the extended family.

13. **4.** If a translator is not present with a client who does not speak English, communication will take more time. The nurse must be creative and patient. Using simple words, gestures, and pictures may prove helpful. Written medical terms will not be effective if the client doesn't understand English. Discussion of one issue at a time does not overcome the language barrier. Rescheduling home visits is not generally acceptable.

14. **2.** Folk remedies are widely accepted practices in the Hispanic-American culture. At times, a combination of folk remedies and Western medicine are utilized. Many Hispanic-American clients will not discuss folk remedies with their physician.

15. **1.** Traditional American Indian health beliefs reflect a bond between person and nature. Health is believed to reflect harmony with the surrounding environment and family. Traditional beliefs focus on wellness, not illness. The body is divided into two halves that are seen as plus and minus or two energy poles, one positive and one negative.

16. **3.** Typical nonverbal behavior of American Indians is quiet listening. Silence is respected and eye contact is considered disrespectful. Communication style is often slow with a low tone of voice and reflection between statements.

17. **1.** During an interview, asking an American Indian to speak louder and repeat responses are seen as rude and disrespectful.

18. **4.** Patrilineal descent is typical of Arab-American families and means a family group consisting of family members on the father's side.

19. **2, 4, 5, 6.** The Arab diet is rich in rice, soup, chicken, and lamb. Fried and canned foods are usually avoided. Pork is prohibited and meat is slaughtered in a specific fashion.

20. **2.** The majority of Arab Americans immigrating to the United States are Muslims. Family members, not friends, are the strongest social unit. Following Islam is the pillar of the Arab-American lifestyle. Meals are often consumed very quickly and in silence.

21. **2.** Generally, Arab-American clients prefer highly technical, even invasive, procedures over noninvasive treatment modalities.

22. **1.** It is typical of the Arab-American culture that immediate pain relief is expected and may be persistently requested. Trying to obtain more information or explaining that the nurse was unaware of the discomfort is not appropriate at this time. Assisting another client should be delegated to another staff member.

23. **1.** Russian-American cultural belief regarding health is very much the idea that one has little or no control over health and illness. Nature, environment, God's will, and eating right have no part in the belief system.

24. 1. Direct eye contact is used and appreciated in the Russian-American culture. Eye contact indicates trustworthiness and honesty. Touch and handshaking are used for formal greetings. Nodding is a gesture of approval.

25. 3. In the case of a terminal illness, a common Russian-American cultural practice is to only disclose the medical condition to nearest relatives. It is believed the client will do better if the client continues to have hope for recovery.

Leadership and Management

■ **ISSUES IN HEALTH CARE DELIVERY**

A. Quality Health Care Issues
1. Types of Health Care Services
   a. Primary health care is the level of services devoted to health promotion and the prevention of illness and/or disability.
   b. Secondary health care is the level of services that focus on detection and early intervention in order to prevent further illness and/or disability.
   c. Tertiary health care services are devoted to restorative and/or rehabilitative services for clients who have chronic and/or irreversible conditions.
2. Population-based Health Care (see Table 2-1)
   a. Description
      Population-based health care focuses on the health care needs of a population of clients rather than individual clients
   b. Management of care is the organized collection of activities designed to meet the needs of the client within a quality and efficient delivery system.
   c. Evidenced-based practice is the delivery of care for clients that is based not only on the clinical expertise of the nurse caregiver but also the recent research findings relative to the client's care needs.
3. Legal and Ethical Issues
   a. Nurse practice acts guide the scope of practice for the professional nurse in each state. State Boards of Nursing monitor the legal practice of professional nurses in each state and nurses must know the state law and use the nurse practice act for guidance and applicable action.

CHAPTER OUTLINE

Issues in Health Care Delivery

Leadership in Professional Nursing

Management in Professional Nursing

Managing Change

Client-care Management

Leading and Managing Client Care

Influence of Power

Time Management in Nursing

NURSING ALERT

Y ou need to be aware when a client is hospitalized for secondary or tertiary care services for a specific health problem, and must continue to provide primary care health promotion services.

NURSING ALERT

N ursing policies concerning clinical practice should be created using evidence-based practice whenever possible.

NURSING ALERT

E very nurse should own a copy of the practice act of the state they practice in and understand how it guides their care.

TABLE 2-1   Features of the New Role of Health Care Management in a Population-Based Health System

Emphasis on the continuum of care

Emphasis on maintaining and promoting wellness

Accountability for the health of defined populations

Differentiation based on ability to add value

Success achieved by increasing the number of covered lives and keeping people healthy

Goal is to provide care at the most appropriate level

Integrated health delivery system

Managers oversee a market

Managers operate service areas across organizational borders

Managers actively pursue quality and continuous improvement

> ## NURSING ALERT
>
> "**S**tandard of care" is usually derived from the state practice act and the body that creates standards of care for nursing specialties. For example, a critical care nurse's standard of care would be judged from standards created by The American Association of Critical Care Nurses.

> ## NURSING ALERT
>
> **G**ood decisions always have ethical principles guiding them, such as justice or autonomy. Poor decisions usually do not have ethical principles guiding them.

    b. Negligence and malpractice are terms that describe a lack of appropriate care as described by the nurse practice act and standards of care.

        1) Negligence is a deviation from the standard of care or carelessness in providing appropriate care that a person of ordinary prudence would exercise in the same circumstances.

        2) Malpractice is the failure of a licensed professional to act in a reasonable and prudent manner with respect to client care needs.

    c. Protective and reporting laws are those laws in each state that require a professional to report incompetent practice, client abuse situations, and professional impairment.

    d. Ethical practice and principles concern the process of making decisions relative to client care and professional practice that is based on distinction of right and wrong concerning knowledge and not just on opinion. Ethical decisions require knowledge, facts, and rules of the situation, options and courses of action that are appropriate, possible consequences, values, and desired goals and outcomes.

■ LEADERSHIP IN PROFESSIONAL NURSING

a. Description

A process in which the leader influences other individuals or groups toward goal achievement. Leadership can be demonstrated in formal or informal roles.

b. Leadership Characteristics

    1. Those attributes and personal characteristics demonstrated by individuals in leadership roles.

NURSING ALERT

N urse managers should be able to describe their leadership style and how the style affects the management process.

2. Vision – Effective leaders focus on the professional, institutional, and purposeful vision that will provide direction toward goal achievement.
3. Passion – The ability to motivate and guide people toward the goal.
4. Integrity – The knowledge of self that demonstrates the values of honesty and maturity and promotes trust among others.

c. Leadership in Action
   1. The traits demonstrated by a leader such as intelligence, self-confidence, determination, integrity, and sociability. Leadership effectiveness is usually demonstrated using one of the following leadership styles:
      a. Autocratic leadership
         Decisions are made by the leader and given directly to others through command and control of others.
      b. Democratic leadership
         Decisions are made by a participatory between the leader and others by delegation of authority to others in the system.
      c. Laissez-faire leadership
         Decision making is deferred to others by a passive and permissive approach.
      d. Transactional leadership
         Decisions may be implicitly defined using the power and formal authority of the organizational position to reward and punish performance
      e. Transformational leadership
         Decisions are explicitly defined through collaboration, consultation, and consensus building among others.

■ MANAGEMENT IN PROFESSIONAL NURSING

a. Description
   A process in which the manager coordinates actions and resources to achieve goals and outcomes for the organization.
b. Management Process
   The activities of planning, organizing, coordinating, and controlling human and physical resources in order to achieve a goal.
   1. POCC
      Acronym describing the role function of the manager involving planning, organizing, coordinating, and controlling.

NURSING ALERT

The one thing that is constant in nursing is change.

NURSING ALERT

C hange agents must have a vision of change and maintain enthusiasm despite any adversity that they may encounter.

2. POSD-CORB
   Acronym describing the role function of the manager involving planning, organizing, staffing, directing, coordinating, reporting, and budgeting.
3. Managerial roles and functions of the nurse
   a. Information processing roles
      Activities used to provide informational needs to others such as monitor, disseminator, director, and spokesperson.
   b. Interpersonal
      Behavorial activities used to motivate and communicate with others such as director, leader, liaison, encourager, and spokesperson.
   c. Decision-making roles
      Activities used to guide and direct goals, plans, and evaluative outcomes such as collaborator, entrepreneur, negotiator, delegator, and communicator.

■ MANAGING CHANGE

1. Change Process
   Process of assessment, planning, implementation, evaluation, and stabilization employed by a leader or manager as a framework to guide planned change in the organization (see Table 2-2)
2. Role of the change agent (see Table 2-3)
   An individual who is responsible for implementing a change project, activity, or process
3. Response to Change
   Behavioral response to the process and outcome of planned change exhibited by those involved in the change project
   a. Innovators
      Those who embrace change and enjoy the challenge.

TABLE 2-2   Comparison Chart of Change Theories and their Uses

Theorist and Year	Lewin (1951)	Lippitt (1958)	Havelock (1973)	Rogers (1983)
Title of Model	Force-Field Model	Phases of Change	Six-Step Change Model	Diffusion of Innovations Theory
Steps in Model (The steps in the models are spaced to indicate their correlation to lewin's model.)	1. Unfreeze 2. Move 3. Refreeze	1. Diagnose problem 2. Assess motivation and capacity for change 3. Assess change agent's motivation and resources 4. Select progressive change objective 5. Chose appropriate role of change agent 6. Maintain change 7. Terminate helping relationship	1. Buildrelationship 2. Diagnoseproblem 3. Acquireresources 4. Choose solution 5. Gain acceptance 6. Stabilization and self-renewal	1. Awareness 2. Interest 3. Evaluation 4. Trial 5. Adoption

Source: Adapted from Introductory Management and Leadership for Nurses *(2nd ed., p. 327) by R. C. Swansburg and R.J. Swansburg (1998), Boston: Jones & Bartlett Publishers.*

CLIENT TEACHING CHECKLIST

t is the RN's responsibility to explain to the client about the care delivery team and each member's role in their care. Clients should understand which member:

- Communicates with the doctors
- Administers pain medications
- Assists with personal care
- Assists with ambulation
- Educates them

TABLE 2-3   Roles and Characteristics of the Change Agent

• Leader of change process	• Communicates change, progress, and feelings
• Manages process and group dynamics	
• Understands feelings of group experiencing the change	• Knowledgeable about the organization
• Maintains momentum and enthusiasm	• Trustworthy
• Maintains vision of change	• Respected
	• Intuitive

   b. Early adopters
      Open and receptive to change but not obsessed with the need to change.
   c. Early majority
      Those that really prefer the status quo but do not want to be left behind by the change event.
   d. Late majority
      Those who adapt to change only after expressing negative feelings and skeptical ideas
   e. Laggards
      Those who prefer tradition and stability; suspicious of the change.
   f. Rejectors
      Those who openly oppose and reject the change project and may hinder the outcome to the point of sabotage.

■ CLIENT-CARE MANAGEMENT

1. Models of Client Care Delivery
   An organizational model for staffing and/or the work of delivery of care to clients.

R egardless of the model of client care delivery used to provide care, it is the RN that is responsible and accountable ultimately for the care provided.

    a. Total Client Care

The registered nurse is responsible for the total care of clients assigned for the shift with or without assistance from a licensed practical nurse (LPN) or an unlicensed assistant personnel (UAP).

    b. Functional Nursing

Nursing care is divided into functional units that are assigned to one of the staff members whose specific duties are compatible with the work to be done.

    c. Team Nursing

Nursing care assignments are given to a team of staff with the responsibility for the entire care of a group of clients. A team leader coordinates and supervises all the care provided by others on the team.

    d. Primary Nursing

The registered nurse is the designated primary care provider for clients with responsibility and accountability for the quality care of the clients assigned on a 24 hour basis.

    e. Client-centered or Client-focused care

Delivery care model where assignment of care is based on client needs rather than staff needs. Care teams are usually interdisciplinary and assigned to a group of clients.

    f. Differentiated nursing practice

Roles, functions, and work of the registered nurse is established according to a set of criteria such as education, clinical experience, competence, and/or certification.

2. Effective Staffing Patterns

    a. Client classification and needs

A system of measurement for describing the nursing workload requirements for a specific client or group of clients based on client care needs.

    b. Nurse Staffing

The process of evaluating the quantity and quality of nursing staff patterns necessary to meet standards of care for clients and to insure quality client outcomes.

    c. Client care outcomes

The process of measuring the effectiveness of client care results based on diagnosis, standards of care, and length of hospital stay, and staffing patterns.

3. Issues in Managing Client Care

    a. Delegation

NURSING ALERT

Delegation is not complete until the RN evaluates the care provided.

TABLE 2-4   Delegation Suggestions for RNs

1. Include all personnel in the delegation process when making assignments.
2. Assess what is to be delegated and identify who would best complete the assignment.
3. Communicate the duty to be performed and identify the time frame for completion. The expectations for personnel should be clear and concise.
4. Avoid removing duties once assigned. This should be considered only when the duty is above the level of the personnel, as when the patient's care is in jeopardy because the patient's status has changed.
5. Evaluate the effectiveness of the delegation of duties, check in frequently, and ask for a feedback report on the outcomes of care delivery.
6. Accept minor variations in the style in which the duties are performed. Individual styles are acceptable as long as the duty is performed correctly within the scope of practice.

     The transferring of authority to perform selected nursing tasks to a competent individual (see Table 2-4)

b. Accountability and responsibility
Accountability is the legal liability for overall nursing care of clients assumed by the nurse. Responsibility includes each nurse's personal obligation, reliability, and dependability to perform client care at an acceptable level based on standards of care.

c. Appropriate Team Delegation
The assignment of client care tasks and duties to personnel who are educated and/or licensed to perform specific quality care tasks. Delegation considerations include potential harm to the client, complexity of care needed, skill at problem solving, predictability of client care outcomes, and need for appropriate, therapeutic interaction. (see Figure 2-1)

d. Conflict Resolution
The ability to resolve conflict or disagreements between other individuals. Sources of conflict include differences of opinion about resources, values, personalities, cultural, and threats to personal self-esteem or organizational position.

e. Conflict Resolution Techniques (see Table 2-5)
Strategies used to resolve the conflict process

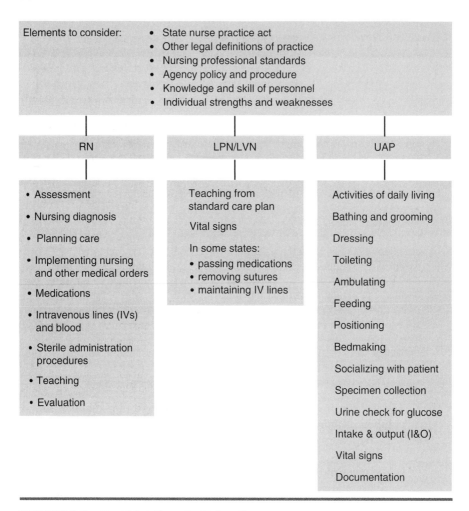

FIGURE 2-1   Considerations in Delegation

TABLE 2-5   Summary of Conflict Resolution Techniques

Conflict Resolution Technique	Advantages	Disadvantages
Avoiding—ignoring the conflict	Does not make a big deal out of nothing; conflict may be minor in comparison to other priorities	Conflict can become bigger than anticipated; source of conflict might be more important to one person or group than others

Accommodating—smoothing or cooperating. One side gives in to the other side	One side is more concerned with an issue than the other side; stakes not high enough for one group and that side is willing to give in	One side holds more power and can force the other side to give in; the importance of the stakes are not as apparent to one side as the other; can lead to parties feeling "used" if they are always pressured to give in
Competing—forcing; the two or three sides are forced to compete for the goal	Produces a winner; good when time is short and stakes are high	Produces a loser; leaves and resentment on losing sides
Compromising—each side gives up something and gains something	No one should win or lose but both should gain something; good for disagreements between individuals	May cause a return to the conflict if what is given up becomes more important than the original goal
Negotiating—high-level discussion that seeks agreement but not necessarily consensus	Stakes are very high and solution is rather permanent; often involves powerful groups	Agreements are permanent, even though each side has gains and losses
Collaborating—both sides work together to develop optimal outcome	Best solution for the conflict and encompasses all important goals to each side	Takes a lot of time; requires commitment to success
Confronting—immediate and obvious movement to stop conflict at the very start	Does not allow conflict to take root; very powerful	May leave impression that conflict is not tolerated; may make something big out of nothing

NURSING ALERT

The antagonist may appear as a negative person on a team, yet they provide valuable insight regarding potential problems.

■ LEADING AND MANAGING CLIENT CARE

A. Effective Team Building
  1. Definition of Teams
     A small group of individuals with a set of skills that compliments each other and who are committed to a common purpose, attainment of goals, desired outcomes, and performance accountability.
  2. Roles within teams are designated or emerge as the purpose and goals of the team become clear. Some individuals take on informal roles to facilitate group effectiveness:
     a. Team leaders usually take on the leadership and management planning, organizing, and creation of the team process.
     b. Coordinators are similar to leaders in that the person is aware of the team goals and direction and assist in keeping the team moving in the right direction.
     c. The mobilizer assist the leader and coordinator in keeping the team energized and interested in goal attainment.
     d. The team questioner is the person who asks the questions, even the ones that others want to ask but avoid, in order to keep the project goals and outcomes clear and concise.
     e. The antagonist is the team member who looks at the situation in the opposite manner as other team members and provides a 'devils advocate' approach to the team process.
     f. The team recorder is the person who records the details of team meetings, process, outcomes, and evaluation.
  3. Roles of dysfunctional team members include those roles and activities that hinder the team progress and goal attainment.
     a. Criticizer's are characterized by resistance to all activities, plans, and goals of the team. If the process is not implemented in a way that they agree with, every action and comments is negative.
     b. Passive team members rarely have input for the team and remain in a quiet, non-contributing mode for fear of rebuttal from other team members.
     c. Detailers are those who get saturated with the details of the team that it is difficult for them to focus on the goal and to see the bigger issues of the team.
     d. Controllers are those team members who try to monopolize the team process by constantly sharing their personal opinions.

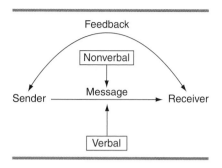

FIGURE 2-2 Basic Communication Model

    e. Team pleasers are those who avoid negative comments and unfavorable decisions in order to please the leader or other group members.

4. Team evaluation is important in order to assess accomplishment of goals and outcomes. Evaluation of the purpose, goals, implementation, outcomes, and team member participation are important to insure future success and outcomes.

Effective Communication Strategies

1. Elements of the communication process (see Figure 2-2)
    a. Communication is the exchange of information, often an interactive process that is influenced by the context
    b. Modes of communication include verbal, nonverbal, and electronic.
2. Nurses must be effective communicators and learn various techniques for enhancing interactions with other nurses, the interdisciplinary health care team, and clients and families. Communication skills include attending, responding, clarifying, and confronting. (see Table 2-6)
3. Because nurses communicate with many diverse individuals and groups in the work setting, skill should also be developed related to the identification of barriers to the communication process. Barriers to effective communication include gender and cultural differences, emotional issues such as stress and anger, incongruent interactive responses, and conflict. (see Table 2-7)

■ INFLUENCE OF POWER

1. Definition of power
The ability to influence others toward goal attainment. Power includes the ability to influence another individual's thinking and/or behavior. For example, the nurse influences the behavior of the client and family during health teaching sessions.

TABLE 2-6   Additional Communication Skills

Skill	Description
Supporting	Siding with another person or backing up another person: "I can see that you would feel that way."
Focusing	Centers on the main point: "So your main concern is . . ."
Open-ended questioning	Allows for patient-directed responses: "How did that make you feel?"
Providing information	Supplies one with knowledge she did not previously have: "It's common for people with pneumonia to be tired."
Using silence	Allows for intrapersonal communication
Reassuring	Restores confidence or removes fear: "I can assure you that tomorrow . . ."
Expressing appreciation	Shows gratitude: "Thank you" or "You are so thoughtful."
Using humor	Provides relief and gains perspective; may also cause harm so use carefully
Conveying acceptance	Makes known that one is capable or worthy: "It's okay to cry."
Asking related questions	Expands the listener's understanding: "How painful was it?"

2. Sources of power relate to factors that allow an individual to influence another and may be formal or informal and conscious or unconscious.
   a. Expert power
      Results from the knowledge and skill that a person ossesses
   b. Legitimate power
      Derived from a position or role that a person holds personally or professionally; associated with some degree of authority as a result of the position
   c. Referent power
      Result of how much others like the individual, respect held for the individual, and trustworthiness of the person.

NURSING ALERT

N urses wield a great deal of power with their clients and must be careful not to use power to coerce a client into doing anything they may not be comfortable with.

TABLE 2-7 Additional Barriers to Communication

Barrier	Description
Offering false reassurance	Promising something that cannot be delivered
Being defensive	Acting as though one has been attacked
Stereotyping	Unfairly categorizing someone based on his or her traits
Interrupting	Speaking before the other has completed her message
Inattention	Not paying attention
Stress	A state of tension that gets in the way of reasoning
Unclear expectations	Ill-defined tasks or duties that make successful completion unlikely

    d. Reward or coercive power

    Derived by the ability a person has to offer reward, punishment, or fear over another individual

    e. Connection power

    The ability of an individual to connect to others and increase their influence by the number of people in the group for which they are associated

    f. Information power

    Derived from a person's ability or position to influence others by the amount and kind of information possessed

    g. Empowerment versus disempowerment in managing client care

       1. Empowerment

       The process of facilitating the participation of others in decision making or a specific activities through instilling the belief that the others have power that needs to be activated

DELEGATION TIP

U sing successful delegation strategies optimizes the nurse's efficiency and helps with effective time management.

    2. Disempowerment
      The process of disabling or diminishing power in an individual or group by influencing the perceived power of that individual or group based on image, opinion, or actions.

■ TIME MANAGEMENT IN NURSING

a. Description
    1. The process or skill of decision making and priority setting that maximizes the most effective and productive use of time.
    2. Nurse managers, nursing staff, and individuals connected to the health care delivery team must understand the larger organizational picture of the unit and/or institution in order to develop achievable goals and use time effectively.
    3. Time management strategies such as knowledge of the overall situation, planning and achieving quality outcomes, and priority setting are important in the overall achievement of client care outcomes. The following order of priority for client care is one example of an approach to time management on a given shift: 1) Life-threatening or potentially life-threatening conditions; 2) Activities that insure safety for clients, families, and co-workers; 3) Activities essential to the plan of care and achievement of optimal client outcomes.
    4. Proper time management is important in decreasing the stress and burnout felt by nurses who are spending numerous hours in the work of managing client care. Strategies to enhance personal time management include scheduling personal time for self, efficient use of periods of downtime, control distractions that interfere with personal time, set attainable personal goals such as exercise, rest, and education.

REVIEW QUESTIONS

1. A family has recently moved to a new metropolitan area and is looking for a health care delivery system that will serve the needs of all family members, including a father who is an older adult and recently had a stroke and is in need of rehabilitative services. The nurse informs the family that which of the following agencies would be the best health care choice?

    1. A home health care service

    2. A university medical center and outpatient services

    3. A suburban community hospital

    4. Health promotion services for the entire family

2. A family selected population-based health care practice of America. The nurse manager teaching this family about the health care services available would include which of the following statements?

    1. "We have an asthma clinic specifically for clients of all ages."

    2. "The major initiative of our care delivery system is restorative care."

    3. "The main advantage to families is that palliative care is the main priority."

    4. "If specialty care is needed, the health care provider will make a referral to a tertiary care system."

3. Based on an understanding of evidence-based client care, the nurse manager should include which of the following instructions for the staff on how to address the home care needs of a group of clients who have had knee replacements?

    1. "I know from experience that these clients will need a concrete exercise plan."

    2. "Most clients exhibit anxiety when describing the stairs within their homes."

    3. "Knee replacement care is complex because of the age of these clients."

    4. "Dietary instructions at home are based on common standards of practice and the most recent research for promoting healing."

4. A new graduate nurse is interviewing for a staff position in a health care delivery system that has agencies in five different states. Which of the following statements indicates that the new nurse understands the legalities of nursing practice, if hired by this company?

    1. "Standards of practice are established by the governing agency, so practice issues will be covered at each agency site."

    2. "A registered nurse license is acknowledged in all of the 50 states without additional paperwork."

3. "The nurse practice act in each state will provide the legal guidelines for professional nursing practice."

4. "The nurse will practice nursing at any of the five agencies based on the nurse practice act in the nurse's home state."

5. After reviewing incident reports for one month, a nurse working in the risk management department at a local health care facility determines which of the following violations of client care is most common?

   1. Physical abuse

   2. Substance abuse

   3. Malpractice actions

   4. Negligence of care

6. Which of the following laws require a nurse to report a peer who is keeping a portion of narcotics ordered for a client?

   1. Reporting laws

   2. Malpractice laws

   3. Jurisdiction laws

   4. Civil court laws

7. Which of the following should the nurse manager include in staff development classes related to ethical decision making?

   1. The practice of ethics is the philosophy of individual opinion and values.

   2. Ethical decisions made in client care are based on the opinion of the client and family.

   3. Ethical decision making is based on knowledge, facts, and a strong commitment to right and wrong.

   4. Ethical decision making in client care can only be made by an interdisciplinary team.

8. The nursing manager on the orthopedic unit evaluates a new staff nurse on the night shift as a born "leader," based on which of the following true leadership qualities?

   1. Having incomplete intake and output records on the night shift was a problem; records have been consistently complete since the new staff nurse arrived

   2. The new staff nurse has scheduled staff journal club discussions once a month to increase current knowledge about client care issues

   3. The new staff nurse always works overtime when asked by the nurse manager

   4. Incomplete shift counts for medications was first noticed by the new staff nurse

9. The astute nurse manager who wishes to empower the nurses on the unit recognizes that strategies must be found to promote their leadership ability. Which of the following supports the nurse manager's knowledge of leadership?

   1. Leadership qualities are demonstrated by those in formal and informal management positions
   2. Nurses at all levels of the organizational chart are not responsible for leadership traits
   3. Leadership characteristics are not measurable on performance appraisals
   4. Only top-level managers have the vision, passion, and integrity to demonstrate leadership

10. The nurse leader who empowers the staff to participate in decision-making activities is exhibiting which of the following leadership styles?

    1. Laissez-faire
    2. Situational
    3. Autocratic
    4. Democratic

11. The nurse describes which of the following leadership models as an integral part of the democratic leadership style?

    1. Transactional
    2. Transformational
    3. Transdepartmental
    4. Transprofessional

12. The management process is incorporated in many job descriptions, such as head nurse, staff nurse, nutritionist, and therapist. Which of the following managerial activities are common to all health care positions?
    Select all that apply:

    [ ] 1. Budgeting
    [ ] 2. Planning
    [ ] 3. Organizing
    [ ] 4. Liaison
    [ ] 5. Coordinating
    [ ] 6. Spokesperson

13. Which of the following are priorities for the nurse manager to incorporate into the nurse manager role of guiding and directing goal achievement?
    Select all that apply:

[   ] **1.** Collaborator

[   ] **2.** Caregiver

[   ] **3.** Negotiator

[   ] **4.** Delegator

[   ] **5.** Communicator

[   ] **6.** Liaison

14. The nurse manager introduces to the staff the new organizational policy and procedural changes for administering blood products. According to Lewin's model for implementing change, which of the following steps of the change process is the nurse manager addressing?

    1. Unfreeze
    2. Move
    3. Refreeze
    4. Evaluate

15. A staff nurse has been assigned to the Standards of Care Committee in which the standard of care for wound care and dressing changes is going to be refined. As an effective change agent, the staff nurse will need to exhibit which of the following characteristics?

    1. Quality interpersonal skills
    2. Respect from clients and families
    3. Expertise in clinical therapeutics
    4. High ethical decision making

16. The nurse manager and staff of a 25-bed surgical unit have decided to change the client care delivery model from primary nursing to team nursing. The nurse manager prepares which of the following statements for the administration that is most appropriate to support this change?

    1. "No transition period will be necessary because all staff have experience working in teams."
    2. "The staffing goal is to have four teams, with a total of 3 to 4 RNs, 2 to 3 LPNs, and 2 nursing assistants for each shift."
    3. "The nursing assistants, who are also senior nursing students, have the knowledge and skill to lead a staffing team."
    4. "The registered nurses on the unit will be assigned 24 hours of responsibility for client care planning."

17. Based on an understanding of the differentiated nursing practice model, nurses on the burn and trauma unit have decided to assign certain client care activities because

1. nurses have client care rounds and discuss differences in client outcomes.

2. there is a pay differential for registered nurses who work overtime.

3. all unit staff are accountable for annual validation of CPR, safety precautions, and client confidentiality guidelines.

4. Batchelor of science nurses (BSN) and master of science nurses (MSN) are expected to plan and implement education and research-based staff development sessions.

18. Based on an understanding of the nurse manager role, the nurse manager was notified at home of a staffing issue for the night shift because

    1. the nurse manager must be an autocratic leader.

    2. the nurse manager has 24-hour, seven-day-a-week accountability for nursing care.

    3. the regular staff members do not have managerial responsibility for problem-solving outcomes of staffing issues.

    4. the nurse manager is responsible for all staff decisions, including staffing changes.

19. Which of the following roles is the charge nurse applying when assigning unlicensed assistive personnel (UAP) to tasks of custodial care, vital sign monitoring, and intake and output measurement for all the clients on the unit?

    1. Delegation

    2. Accountability

    3. Responsibility

    4. Outcome measurement

20. The nurse manager incorporates which of the following functional roles of the team members when planning to conduct a class on effective team building and group process?

    1. There will always be one person who wants to dominate the discussion using personal examples

    2. Every group needs a person in the role of creator, coordinator, and record keeper

    3. An effective team always rallies around the leadership traits demonstrated by the group or team spokesperson

    4. Some teams are motivated to get the job done in spite of dysfunctional behavior of a few team members

21. The communication process is essential to the leader or manager role and to the role of the manager of client care. It is essential for all managers,

including the manager of client care, to be effective communicators. The nurse who effectively analyzes the communication process understands that messages are

1. synchronous and asynchronous.
2. coded and encoded.
3. verbal and nonverbal.
4. native and foreign.

22. Which of the following communication skills should the nurse include when planning to manage client care? Select all that apply:

[ ] 1. Observation
[ ] 2. Attending
[ ] 3. Teaching
[ ] 4. Responding
[ ] 5. Clarifying
[ ] 6. Focusing

23. The nurse should consider which of the following sources of power to be most effective within an organization?

1. Expert
2. Referent
3. Connection
4. Legitimate

24. The nurse should include which of the following in the discharge instructions given to a client who was recently diagnosed with diabetes mellitus to promote dietary compliance?

1. Empowerment
2. Authority
3. Connectedness
4. Charisma

25. The nurse manager called a meeting with one of the unit team leaders because clients have complained that they are not receiving their medication on time. The nurse manager should include which of the following good time management strategies during the meeting with the unit team leader?

1. The nurse manager wants all team leaders to take the first hour of each shift to set client care priorities
2. The nurse manager realizes that time management strategies are unrealistic when staffing is too low

3. All team leaders must look at the overall work to be done and set appropriate priorities

4. Optimal outcomes can only be achieved by implementing essential physical tasks

26. The charge nurse must transfer a client from a medical-surgical unit to a maternity unit in order to make a bed available. It would be most appropriate for the charge nurse to transfer which client?

   1. A 55-year-old client with tonic-clonic seizures

   2. A 22-year-old client with a gastrointestinal bleed on a vasopressin (Pitressin) drip

   3. A 40-year-old client who had a knee replacement with a continuous motion device

   4. A 30-year-old mastectomy client who will be discharged

ANSWERS AND RATIONALES

1. **2.** Tertiary health care services include restorative and rehabilitative services for clients of all ages. A university medical center with outpatient services is best equipped to deliver care across the continuum for this family. A home health care service, suburban community, and health promotion services for the entire family are limited to a specific level of care.

2. **1.** Population-based health care practice is the development, provision, and evaluation of multidisciplinary health care services to population groups experiencing an increased risk in partnership with consumers of health care and the community, in order to improve the health of the community and its diverse population groups. Population-based care is a managed care approach for a specific group of clients, not just individuals. The goal of care in a population-based system is to maintain and promote wellness, not restorative care. Specialty care and palliative care can be a part of the services, but may not be the priority; nor is referral necessary to a larger system.

3. **4.** Evidenced-based practice is a combination of knowledge and expertise in clinical practice, as well as the most recent research findings with each specific client. While clients usually understand the exercise plan needed to strengthen overall muscle and joints, anxiety can be minimized with teaching and practice dealing with steps. Knee replacement care is complex, but the age of the client is not relevant. Dietary instructions, such as increase protein, are important for healing following a knee replacement.

4. 3. Nurse practice acts may differ from state to state. The state board of nursing for each state monitors the legal practice of nursing in each state. While standards of care may be policy at each agency, they do not override the standards outlined in the nurse practice act for each agency's state. Once an RN license has been obtained, reciprocity to practice in other states must be granted by each state board.

5. 4. Negligence is the most common violation of client care in health care facilities. Negligence is a deviation from the appropriate standard of care, usually due to carelessness. Physical abuse, substance abuse, and malpractice actions are all criminal acts and occur less frequently.

6. 1. Reporting laws in each state require a professional to report incompetent practice, client abuse, and professional impairment. Malpractice laws, jurisdiction laws, and civil court laws may vary from state to state.

7. 3. Making ethical decisions requires skill in analyzing knowledge, facts, rules of care, and a strong personal distinction between what is right and wrong in a specific client situation. Opinion is not the driving force in decision making. Ethical decision making in client care made by an interdisciplinary team is ultimately possible when ethics committees meet to discuss individual client cases. It is important to remember that every nurse practices as an individual professional and incorporates ethical decision making into everyday practice.

8. 2. Knowing the importance of keeping up-to-date on practice issues and having the confidence to implement a strategy to discuss client care issues as a new staff member both demonstrate leadership quality in this staff nurse.

9. 1. Leadership qualities and an ability to influence others to achieve goals can be exhibited by any employee in an organization. Individuals with good management skills may not demonstrate leadership ability.

10. 4. Democratic leaders seek participation in decision-making activities by all levels of staff affected at the unit level. Laissez-faire leadership is a passive and permissive style of leadership that defers decision making. An autocratic leadership style involves decision making that is centralized with the leader making decisions and using power to command and control others. Situational leadership confirms that there is not one best leadership style, but rather that effective leadership is matched to the group's level of task-relevant readiness.

11. 1. Transformational leadership theory includes explicitly seeking collaboration, consultation, and consensus building among team members. Transactional leadership model is aligned with transactional leadership. Transdepartmental and transprofessional are strategies, not

leadership models, for gathering information across departments within an organization or within the profession as a whole.

● 12. **2, 3, 5.** Managers of human resources, client care, and other health-related disciplines include role functions of planning, organizing, and coordinating client care activities. Not all personnel have the responsibilities of budgeting, department liaison, or director and spokesperson.

● 13. **1, 3, 4, 5.** While functioning as a caregiver and liaison is possible, the functions that are the priority for the nurse manager are collaborator, negotiator, delegator, and communicator. Nurse managers may have to assume the duties of caregiver in certain circumstances, but usually they do not have a client care assignment. The liaison role is usually carried out by the nursing staff, on behalf of the client. The nurse manager would function as spokesperson to speak on behalf of the staff of a department.

14. **1.** The first step for implementing change, or unfreezing, is to assist others to understand the need for change and the steps necessary to implement the change. Communication and information sharing are essential in this step. Actual implementation of the change and accepting the change as the standard of care are activities that occur with moving and refreezing. Evaluating is necessary for overall quality management, but is not a part of the change process as described by Lewin's change theory.

15. **1.** Although respect from clients and families, expertise in clinical therapeutics, and high ethical decision making are admirable for the staff nurse, the change process related to procedure of wound care and dressing changes will need to be discussed hospitalwide, unit by unit, utilizing quality interpersonal skills. Teaching and information sharing are essential when a change affects so many people, and these require quality interpersonal skills.

16. **2.** A staffing goal of having four teams with a total of 3 to 4 RNs, 2 to 3 LPNs, and 2 nursing assistants is the best staffing option for implementing care based on flexibility and acuity of client care for a 25-bed unit. Transition in staffing and operational issues will be necessary even if all staff members have previously worked using a team nursing model. Assuming that all nursing assistants are senior nursing students is not a legally sound staffing assignment. Assigning a registered nurse to be responsible for 24-hour client care is indicative of a primary nursing model.

17. **4.** Expectations to plan and implement education and research-based staff development sessions by bachelor of science nurses (BSN) and master of science nurses (MSN) are best, considering that the assignment of educational sessions is based on the education level of the nursing staff. Differentiated practice includes the assignment of duties based on education level, competence, and certification. Nurses who have client care rounds, staff nurses who work overtime, and unit staff members who

are held accountable for violation of unit requirements all require nurses to do similar activities regardless of education, clinical expertise, and competence levels.

18. **2.** The nurse manager has 24-hour, seven-day-a-week accountability for nursing care. Nursing staff members are participative decision makers because of their position in the organization. Staff members should have input into the overall decision-making process.

19. **1.** Delegation is the assignment of tasks to others who are competent and skilled to perform them. Accountability and responsibility are qualities that all caregivers must demonstrate, regardless of level of position. While the unlicensed assistive personnel (UAP) may collect data to carry out a nursing task, a nurse at a higher education level would be responsible for the overall evaluation and reporting.

20. **2.** Every group needs a person in the role of creator and coordinator as well as a record keeper. This description contains the functional roles of members of a team. A dominator is a person who wants to dominate. Some teams always rally around the leadership traits of a member of the group or team, but it takes all team members working together collaboratively to be an effective team. Some teams are motivated to get the job done in spite of the dysfunctional behavior of a few team members, but to be a more effective group all team members need to work together.

21. **3.** The most effective communication process includes both verbal and nonverbal cues. The terms synchronous and asynchronous and coded and encoded describe communication concepts within computer technology. Native and foreign describe language as being one's first, or native, language or a language learned later, that is, a foreign language.

22. **2, 4, 5, 6.** Facilitating communication requires more than verbal and nonverbal cues. Strategies to enhance understanding of the message communicated by the client and others will assist the nurse to provide quality, accurate feedback. Communication skills that should be used to manage client care include attending, responding, clarifying, and focusing. Observation and teaching are skills needed by the nurse in planning client care, but are not necessarily strategies for accurate and effective communication.

23. **4.** Legitimate power is the minimum source of power, derived by merely holding a position of authority. Expert, referent, and connection are all sources of power that are derived in ways other than by holding a position. Expert power is power derived from the knowledge and skills the nurse possesses. Referent power, also known as charismatic power, is power conferred by others, based on their respect and liking for an individual, group or organization. Connection power is the connection between nurses having power, such as networking between positions of authority.

24. **1.** Empowerment involves the ability to facilitate the participation of others to action and appropriate decision making. In the case of a client with diabetes mellitus and the need for dietary compliance, the nurse facilitates empowerment and compliance by teaching the client what the correct choices are. Authority and charisma do not ensure compliance. For some older clients, these traits of authority and charisma might be negative influences. Connectedness is a possible influence on the client, but because it would require that the nurse connect often with the client to assess compliance, it would not be a realistic motivator.

25. **3.** All team leaders must look at the overall work to be done and set appropriate priorities. Time management can be accomplished by knowing the overall needs of the clients and then setting appropriate priorities. Team leaders who take the first half hour of every shift to set priorities are lacking time management skills; the tasks could be handled by efficient shift reporting. During a nursing shortage, time management skills are essential and should be realistic.

26. **1.** Obstetrical nurses would have the appropriate knowledge and skills to care for a client having seizures because they routinely care for pregnant women who have hypertension and experience eclampsia (seizures).

3

Ethical Issues

ETHICS

A. Description
1. Ethics is a way of examining, understanding, and making decisions about what actions are right or wrong according to societal norms, and accepted morality
2. Responsibility of all nurses to recognize ethical issues and apply ethical principles and methods of ethical decision making on a daily basis
3. An ethical issue or dilemma arises when there is a decision to be made but it is not clear what may be right or wrong due to reasonable arguments and conflicting moral principles or rules for either action
4. Ethical theories guide the way a nurse examines a situation
5. Professions such as nursing develop codes of conduct to communicate the values of the profession, and reinforce and guide ethical behavior among its members in order to demonstrate its commitment to the trust granted it by society
6. Ethic's committees exist to provide consultation and guidance to healthcare professionals faced with complex ethical dilemmas however, their purpose is not to resolve the dilemma

PHYSIOLOGICAL BASIS UPON WHICH TO ESTABLISH ETHICAL THEORIES

1. Naturalism
   a. View of moral judgment that sees ethics as dependent upon human nature and psychology
   b. Explains differences in moral codes to social conditions and at the same time suggesting a basic congruence to the possession by underlying psychological tendencies suggesting there is a universality in moral judgment

NURSING ALERT

T he American Nurses Association Code of Ethics for Nurses helps nurses guide their practice and conduct in an ethically correct manner.

    c. Individuals or a group of individuals make judgments based on feelings about certain actions in certain situations resulting in most individual's judgments being much the same in situations that are the same

2. Rationalism
    a. Opposite view of naturalism
    b. Believes that feelings although viewed as similar in people may not be similar at all
    c. The foundation of their belief is based on absolute truth that is not dependent upon human nature
    d. They believe that values in ethics have an origin in the nature of the universe or God that may become known through the process of reasoning
    e. Have a belief that there are truths about the world that are not only true but universal and superior to the information received by the senses
    f. Perceive moral rules as true

■ ETHICAL THEORIES

A. Description
    1. An ethical theory is a framework that guides a nurse's reflection on the dilemma
B. Types
    1. Utilitarianism
        a. The right action is that which yield the greatest good for the greatest number of people
        b. Gives equal weights to all parties involved in the dilemma
        c. Based on the principle of utility or achieving the maximum value out of the action
        d. ''Act utilitarianism'' – moral rules can be suspended in some circumstances if they do not maximize the greatest good for the greatest number
        e. ''Rule utilitarianism'' – moral rules may not be suspended because doing so does not lead to the greatest good in the long run
    2. Kantianism
        a. Categorical imperative – the action is right if such an action is willed to become a universal law

NURSING ALERT

N o matter what theory of ethics a nurse utilizes, each provides a framework to help nurses with an ethical dilemma.

  b. Persons must be treated as ends and never as only a means to an end
  c. Correct actions are based on one's obligations to others
  d. May be called deontology or formalism
3. Virtue or Character Ethics
  a. Believes an individual is capable of learning and practicing through the repetition of acts
  b. The virtue is habituated
  c. May be used to nurture or predict character in individuals

■ ETHICAL PRINCIPLES
A. Description
  1. Make up principle-based or common-morality theory
  2. Incorporate concepts from other theories
  3. Must be balanced against each other when making an ethical decision
B. Autonomy
  1. Self-rule and freedom to act
  2. Opposite of paternalism
  3. Nurses must safeguard client's autonomy by providing information and protecting clients from controlling constraints so they may use their freedom effectively
  4. A client's autonomy should be respected as long as in so doing it does not pose a greater harm to others
  5. May be suspended if a client is incapable of self-rule such as infants or suicidal clients
  6. Limited autonomy to make decisions about meals and some care should be granted even to clients who are not deemed competent to make legal or other types of decisions
  7. Informed consent - providing sufficient information and guidance to the client so that they may accept or decline a procedure or participation in research is based on this principle
C. Beneficence
  1. Doing good or to benefit others
  2. What one ought to do such as preventing or removing harm, or promoting good
  3. Required to do good based on the relationship between parties such as the nurse-client relationship

    4. Usually overridden by respect for autonomy such as the nurse respecting the client's right to autonomy to choose over their obligation to do good

D. Nonmaleficence
    1. Obligation not to cause intentional harm
    2. Must be obeyed regardless of relationship
    3. Provide reasons for legal prohibition of certain activities

E. Justice
    1. Fairness and appropriate distribution of resources
    2. Relate to health care policy and social programs

F. Confidentiality
    1. Requires nondisclosure of private or secret information that one is entrusted with
    2. The basis of this principle is based on the oaths of nursing
    3. Not divulging information shared in confidence
    4. Clients have a right to expect that their private medical information will not be shared with anyone other than those needing it to provide their care

G. Fidelity
    1. Relates to the concept of faithfulness and the practice of keeping promises and loyalty with in the nurse-client relationship
    2. Promise-keeping and trust
    3. Loyalty to the client
    4. Client abandonment is an example of breaching this rule

DELEGATION TIP

W hen delegating tasks, you must remind the assistive personnel that any medical information given to help guide care for the client must be kept in confidence.

H. Veracity
  1. Truthtelling
  2. Obligation to tell the truth is based on respect for others
  3. Vital to maintenance of the therapeutic relationship

■ ETHICAL DECISION MAKING

A. Description
  1. Multiple frameworks exist by which to systematically evaluate the ethical theories and principles relevant and in conflict in a given ethical dilemma
  2. Nurses should choose and use ethical decision-making tools to guide them in their actions
  3. Hospital ethic's committees should be utilized by nurses whenever there is conflict over resolution of an ethical dilemma

■ RELATIONSHIP BETWEEN ETHICS AND THE LAW

A. Description
  1. Ethics is the foundation of the law
  2. Law is the system of rules of action or conduct that determines the behavior of individuals in respect to relationships with others and the government
  3. Because laws are created by individuals ethics and law are not always congruent
  4. Laws fall into public or private realms and are constitutional, statutory, or administrative
    a. Constitutional law is based on the Constitution and takes precedence over all other laws
    b. Legislative law also known as statutory law is developed at the state or federal legislatures
    c. Administrative law consists of legal powers given to administrative agencies by legislative bodies and the rules the agencies implement to carry out those policies such as the State Boards of Nursing
    d. Common law also known as case law is a type of law based on previous court decisions

- The nature of the health concern and prognosis if nothing is done.
- Description of all treatment options, even those that the health care provider does not favor or cannot provide.
- The benefits, risks, and consequences of the various treatment alternatives, including noninterventions.

FIGURE 3-1   Content of Informed Consent

B. Types of Law
  1. Public law is the relationship between individuals and the government
  2. Private law is the relationship between individuals
  3. Contract law deals with the obligations and rights of individuals who make contracts such as an implied contract between the nurse and the client to deliver safe and competent
  4. Tort law is an injury or wrongful act that a individual suffers because of another individual's intentional or unintentional actions involving the concepts of malpractice and negligence making it the division of law the nurse is most familiar with
     a. Negligence is the omission of an act that another reasonable individual would do in the same situation such as a nurse who fails to wipe up a water spill on the floor that the client had spilled
     b. Malpractice is a type of negligence in which there is a professional misconduct due to a lack of professional skill that results in harm to the client such as a medication error

▉ LEGAL ISSUES

A. Informed consent
  1. Provides legal protection to a client's right to personal autonomy such as a client who may choose a course of action regarding the plan for their health care
  2. Includes disclosure and essential information that will allow a client to make an informed decision about their care (see Figure 3-1)
  3. The client has the opportunity to accept or refuse the proposed treatment
  4. Although treatment recommendations may be given, the client's consent must be free of coercion or manipulation by the health care provider
  5. Before witnessing a consent, the nurse should assess if the client has a clear understanding of a proposed procedure or needs further explanation such as explaining the benefits and risks of surgery

B. Advance Directives
   1. Directions that are implemented or withheld or a designation of someone who will act as a surrogate in making decisions for an individual who loses their decisions makeing capability
   2. May be considered a form of informed consent for future interventions such as life and death issues when the client is unable to make those decisions
   3. Patient Self-Determination Act requires hospitals, nursing homes, health maintenance organizations, and home care agencies to provide written information to adult clients regarding their rights to make decisions about their health care decisions
   4. Nurses have the responsibility to make sure clients have the right to complete advance directives and to ensure that their wishes are carried through when the time comes
   5. The nurses needs to know their state's statutes that guide advance directives
   6. The nurse has the responsibility to understand the client's wishes for advance directives and to communicate those wishes to other members of the health care team
   7. A client who is admitted with an advance directive does not necessarily mean that the client is a do not resuscitate (DNR)
C. Do Not Resuscitate Orders
   1. Directions to withhold cardiopulmonary resuscitation that must be written and placed in a client's medical record
   2. Whether to initiate CPR requires professional, ethical, legal, and institutional considerations
   3. The general principle for when to implement CPR is that it should be initiated unless it would be futile to do so or unless the physician has specific orders not to do so
   4. The DNR order should be immediately documented in a client's medical record stating why the order was written, who gave the consent, who was present for the discussion, if the client was competent to give consent, and the time frame for the DNR order
   5. Prior to making an informed consent, the client and the family should be informed about the client's condition and prognosis
   6. A DNR order requires the nurse to be focused on comfort interventions and to serve as a support system
   7. Although obtaining a DNR order, the nurse needs to be informed of each client's orders

1. A student nurse asks the nurse, "Why did my advisor recommend an ethics class for me?" Which of the following is the best response by the nurse?

    1. "It is the responsibility of nurses to recognize ethical dilemmas in clinical situations."

    2. "Ethics must be learned in order to obey the law."

    3. "You must have misunderstood because nurses do not have to study ethics."

    4. "You may find studying ethics interesting."

2. The nurse tells another nurse that which of the following best describes the purpose of the American Nurses Association Code for Nurses?

    1. To communicate the values of the profession

    2. To defend the actions of nurses in lawsuits

    3. To develop the good character of nurses

    4. To help recognize nurses for their ethical behavior

3. Which of the following is the best example of an ethical dilemma faced by the nurse?

    1. Deciding whether or not to place a client in a private room

    2. Deciding whether or not to tell a client about the client's diagnosis

    3. Deciding the order in which staff members should take their breaks

    4. Deciding whether or not to ask another nurse to care for a very complex patient

4. A nurse is asked to keep the client's cancer progression from family members until after a daughter's wedding next week, so as not to distract from this important day. This will require the nurse to withhold information from the client's spouse and daughter who accompanied the client to the clinic. Which of the following action by the nurse best demonstrates the theory of utilitarianism?

    1. The nurse tells the client that truth telling is an ethical rule that nurses must uphold and asks the client to reconsider this request

    2. The nurse tells the client's spouse about the disease progression in secret, making the spouse promise not to tell the client

    3. The nurse does as the client wishes and keeps the diagnosis from the family until after the wedding

    4. The nurse informs the client that sharing the diagnosis will facilitate coping and that the family must be told today in the clinic

5. A nurse is asked to keep the client's cancer progression from family members indefinitely. This will require the nurse to withhold information from the client's spouse, who frequently accompanies the client to the clinic. Which of the following actions by the nurse best demonstrates the theory of Kantianism?

   1. The nurse persuades the client to tell the family because it is the right thing to do

   2. The nurse considers multiple ethical principles and supports the client in telling the family, as should be done universally in such a situation

   3. The nurse remembers the ethical rule of truth telling and decides to tell the client's spouse in secret

   4. The nurse considers multiple ethical principles and does not tell the family, because client confidentiality is of primary importance

6. After the physician explains the surgery to the client, the nurse provides the client with information about surgery, answers the client's questions, and allows the client to agree or refuse to have surgery. Which of the following ethical principles is best described by the nurse's actions?

   1. Nonmaleficence

   2. Beneficence

   3. Truth telling

   4. Autonomy

7. The nurse informs a young, healthy client that the scarce amount of flu vaccine will be given to older clients and those with immunosuppressed responses first. Which of the following ethical principles is best described by the nurse's statement?

   1. Beneficence

   2. Autonomy

   3. Justice

   4. Nonmaleficence

8. The nurse chooses to delay taking a break so that pain medication could be administered on time rather than making the client wait until the nurse's break is complete. Which of the following ethical principles is best described by the nurse's action?

   1. Beneficence

   2. Justice

   3. Nonmaleficence

   4. Autonomy

9. A mentally ill client with an order for a general diet requests a vegetarian meal. Which of the following actions by the nurse best demonstrates the nurse's understanding of the principle of autonomy?

1. Tell the client that a vegetarian meal cannot be substituted for a general diet

2. If necessary, obtain an order from the physician for a vegetarian meal; otherwise, provide a vegetarian meal per the client's request

3. Contact the client's family and obtain their consent to provide a vegetarian meal to the client

4. Contact the client's medical power of attorney for permission to make a diet change

10. The nurse returns to the client's room in exactly four hours to administer the next dose of pain medication as promised. Which of the following ethical rules is best demonstrated by the nurse?

1. Justice

2. Nonmaleficence

3. Fidelity

4. Confidentiality

ANSWERS AND RATIONALES

1. **1.** Recognizing ethical dilemmas is the responsibility of all nurses, as well as physicians. Ethical behavior is a component of both law and religion, but knowledge of these areas does not render studying ethics unnecessary.

2. **1.** Ethical codes of professions, such as nursing, are developed to communicate the values of the profession and to guide ethical behavior among its members. The code cannot make nurses behave ethically, nor is its purpose to defend nursing to other professionals or in legal matters.

3. **2.** An ethical dilemma exists when the nurse must make a decision about what is right or wrong, but there are conflicting moral principles or rules with any action taken. While deciding on room assignments and breaks are decisions nurses make daily, these are not ethical dilemmas. Nurses should use good judgment and refuse being assigned to clients whose care is too complex for their training. Withholding information about a diagnosis potentially brings up conflicting issues of veracity, fidelity, and beneficence and is, therefore, an ethical dilemma.

4. **3.** Utilitarianism is a moral theory that holds an action is judged as good or bad in relation to the consequences. It attempts to maximize the greatest good for the greatest number, giving equal weight to all parties involved. The nurse must consider the feelings of the client, family members, and all

others potentially affected by the sharing of the diagnosis. According to the theory of utilitarianism, the nurse must suspend the principle of veracity in order to fulfill the wishes of the client and sustain the happiness that is sure to come to the family members through the wedding celebration. While obtaining support from one's family does support coping, there is no indication that the client is not coping well at this time, and there will be time for coping after the wedding. The nurse must also consider the obligation to uphold the client's confidentiality.

5. **2.** Kantianism, also called deontology, is based on the rationalist view that the rightness or wrongness of an act depends on the nature of the act. The theory of Kantianism uses the categorical imperative to test actions. This imperative states that a person should act as one would wish everyone to act (as if it were a universal law) in that situation. It also says that persons should be treated as ends rather than as means to an end. Pressuring the client treats the client as a means to the end, with which the nurse feels more comfortable and avoids conflict. Keeping the disease progression secret supports the client in treating the spouse as a means to an end by being dishonest. Neither truth telling nor confidentiality alone always applies under this theory, but what is important is a consideration of how one ought to behave if one's actions were to become a universal law. Since sharing the cancer diagnosis with the family is known to support coping of the client and family, it would be generally accepted to support this behavior in most situations in order to uphold principles of beneficence, autonomy, and rule of veracity. Therefore, the nurse should not take the responsibility of telling, but should provide guidance, education, and support to the client's behavior of telling.

6. **4.** The principle of autonomy is upheld when sufficient information and guidance are provided by the nurse so that the client may freely give informed consent. Beneficence is doing good, while nonmaleficence is not doing harm. Truth telling is an ethical rule rather than a principle, and relates to the nurse's obligation to be truthful out of respect for the client.

7. **3.** Equitable distribution of resources is described by the principle of justice. Beneficence is doing good, and nonmaleficence is not doing harm. Autonomy is providing the freedom to act.

8. **1.** Beneficence is described as doing what one ought to do to promote good. Nonmaleficence is not causing intentional harm. Justice is the equitable distribution of resources. Autonomy is upholding a client's right to make informed choices.

9. **2.** Limited autonomy, such as what type of meal to eat, may be granted to those clients who are not deemed competent for other medical decisions.

Neither the client's family nor the power of attorney needs to be contacted to make a diet change, even if they make other types of medical decisions for the client.

10. 3. Justice and nonmaleficence are ethical principles dealing with fair distribution of services and doing no harm. These are principles, not rules. Confidentiality is an ethical rule emphasizing the importance of respecting the client's right to privacy of information. Fidelity is the rule demonstrated by this nurse by keeping the promise made and returning with the pain medication.

4

Legal and Ethical Issues for the Older Adult

■ LEGAL ISSUES OF THE OLDER ADULT

A. Description
1. Registered nurses practicing with older adults and their families need knowledge of basic laws and must be sure their practice falls within legal boundaries
2. Clients and families may ask for advice about wills and advance directives
3. Nurses must be advocates for the older adults and protect their rights.

B. Legal risks for nursing practice with the older adult
1. Situations which increase the risk of liability for a nurse include
   a. Working with insufficient resources
   b. Failing to follow policies and procedures
   c. Taking shortcuts
   d. Working when physically or emotionally exhausted
2. When the standard of care for a given group such as older adults or situation is not followed by the nurse, negligence or malpractice may be charged
   a. Administering the incorrect dosage of a medication and the client suffers harm
   b. Identifying a serious client behavior such as respiratory distress and not informing the primary health care provider in a timely manner
   c. Not providing for safety of a client such as pouring liquid soap for wound cleansing into a medicine cup and leaving it at the bedside of a client who is confused and the client drinks it
   d. Failing to turn an immobile client for an entire shift and the client gets a pressure ulcer
   e. Placing a food tray outside the reach of a client who is unable to self-feed
3. The following conditions must be present for malpractice to exist:
   a. There was a failure to perform at the level of the standard of care
   b. Physical or mental injury resulted to the client or a violation of the client's right resulting from the nurse's negligence.

DELEGATION TIP

R Ns working in long-term facilities delegate care to numerous licensed practical nurses, nurse's aids, and assistive personnel. Although the responsibility is shared among team members, the accountability that the appropriate standard of care is given to clients ultimately rests with the RN.

4. Acts that could result in legal liability
   a. Assault
      A deliberate threat or attempt to harm another person that the person believes could be carried through such as telling a client that if they doesn't eat their breakfast they won't be given any lunch.
   b. Battery
      Unconsented touching of the client in a socially impermissible way or carrying through an assault such as performing a procedure without consent.
   c. Defamation of character
      An oral or written communication to a third party that damage's a person's reputation such as when transferring a client from one facility to another and writing on the transfer papers "He's a dirty old man. Watch out!"
   d. False imprisonment
      Unlawful restraint or detention of a person such as physically preventing a client who is competent from leaving a facility or even telling a client that they will be tied to their bed or locked up if they try to leave.
   e. Fraud
      Willful and intentional misrepresentation intended to produce a unlawful gain such as overcharging a client for services in which older adults tend to be trusting and easy prey for fraud from strangers, acquaintances or unscrupulous family members.
   f. Invasion of privacy
      Invading the right of a client to personal privacy such as an unwanted publicity such as putting a picture of the client in the paper without permission, releasing a medical record to unauthorized persons, giving client information to an inappropriate person or agency (allowing a student nurse who is not assigned to a client to look at that client's chart), or having one's private affairs made public (discussing a client in a public place where the discussion can be heard). Federal regulations, as well as the state govern the client's privacy

> ### DELEGATION TIP
>
> The RN must assure that assistive personnel have a practical understanding of these legal concepts to avoid legal liability. These terms should be described as they relate to care and what activities to circumvent to prevent legally precarious situations.

    g. Larceny

      Unlawful taking of a client's possession such as taking the client's personal items including candy, jewelry or monies from a nursing home resident or clothing which is given to another resident to wear

    h. Negligence

      Omission or commission of an act that departs from acceptable and reasonable standards of practice such as failing to monitor a clients bowel movement pattern and the client develops an impaction

    i. Malfeasance

      Committing an unlawful or improper act such as a nurse performing surgery on a client's leg ulcer

    j. Misfeasance

      Performing an act improperly such as a nurse starting a prescribed intravenous infusion in the foot of a client with impaired circulation

    k. Nonfeasance

      Failure to take proper action such as not notifying the primary health care provider of a serious change in the client's status

    l. Malpractice

      Failure to abide by the standards of practice of the nursing profession such not checking if the nasogastric tube is in the stomach before administering the tube feeding

    m. Criminal negligence

      Disregard protecting the safety of another person such as allowing a client who is confused and receiving oxygen to have access to cigarettes and a lighter in an unsupervised situation

Informed Consent

1. Description

    a. Consent is a voluntary act by which a person agrees to have something done to them by someone else

    b. Informed consent is a process by which a client knows the reason for the proposed treatment as well as it's benefits and risks and is implied by signing a consent form

---

CLIENT TEACHING CHECKLIST

When a client has been appointed a legal guardian, the guardian should know:

- Their legal responsibility to the client
- The medical and psychosocial issues the client may experience
- Who to contact if they have questions regarding their role as guardian

---

NURSING ALERT

If an older client has a legal guardian, you should explain the procedure to both the client and the guardian, but obtain the actual consent from the guardian.

---

   c. Clients have the right to know the full implications of procedures and make an independent decision as to whether or not the procedure should be preformed. Obtaining an informed consent in the older adult may be difficult if the client has been declared legally incompetent and has a guardian. Clients who have a fluctuating level of mental function or who are not fully able to comprehend are incapable of giving legal consent. Consent must be obtained from the legal guardian.

   d. Protects the client's right to self-determination

   e. If in doubt about whether written consent is necessary in a given situation, it is best to err on the side of safety by obtaining witnessed consent from the client if the client is competent or from the legal guardian.

   f. If the client or guardian refuses a prescribed procedure it is useful to have the responsible party sign a release stating that consent is denied and that the risks associated with refusing consent are understood such as refusing to receive a prescribed influenza vaccination.

Competency

1. Description

   a. Competency is the client's ability to make rational decisions regarding care

   b. The client must be able to make decisions voluntarily.

   c. The client has access to information relevant to the health problem and to related decisions.

NURSING ALERT

A lternative methods and techniques should be attempted and documented prior to obtaining an order for restraints.

    d. The client must be legally declared incompetent before a designated guardian has the right to make health care decisions.

    e. Advance directives signed by a client who is competent and witnessed provides for a surrogate to make health care decisions if the client is no longer able to do so

Supervision of Other Health Care Team members

1. Description

    a. The registered nurse has the responsibility to supervise the care which is delegated to other licensed and unlicensed personnel.

    b. This supervision may be direct or indirect as identified in the nurse practice laws of the legal jurisdiction.

Medication administration

1. Description

    a. Each legal jurisdiction identifies who may administer medications to not only all clients but also to vulnerable older adults. The registered nurse caring for older adults has the responsibility to know the prescribed medications, adverse reactions, interactions and contraindications even if a licensed or unlicensed personnel such as a medication aide administers the medications in the nursing home or a family member in the home.

Restraints

1. Description

    a. The Omnibus Budget Reconciliation Act (OBRA) designates the rights of the client and the responsibilities of the providers of health care regarding the use of either physical or chemical restraints or both

    b. The older adult has a right to the safest and least restrictive environment.

    c. Other methods to avoid restraints should be used such as looking in on the client whenever passing the client's room or keeping the bed in the lowest possible position

    d. Restraints are legal only if they are used to protect the client or protect others from harm

    e. If the nurse applied restraints in an emergency situation to a client who is combative or unruly, the nurse must obtain an order immediately

f. A legal "order" from a licensed prescriber, such as a physician or nurse practitioner, is necessary for physical restraints of a client. This includes the use of side rails, a lap belt restraint, or a chest restraint.

g. The use of a chemical agent, such as a sedative, for restraint of the client must also require a legal "order".

h. A restraint such as bed rails should be agreed to in writing by a client who is competent or by the legal guardian.

i. Documentation of the client behavior, need for the restraint for safety, monitoring the client frequently and removal of the restraint is must be preformed requently and according to agency policy

Telephone orders

1. Description
   a. Medical orders from a physician are frequent in the care of the older adult whether in home health or long term care.
   b. The possibility of error is great with a verbal order. Repetition and clarification of the order is necessary to prevent errors.
   c. Agency policy will identify if a registered nurse may take a verbal order from the physician's office personnel.

"No-code" orders

1. Description
   a. Each legal jurisdiction will identify the scope of medical orders which indicate "no code" status for a client.
   b. In general, if the client does not have advance directives all measures will be used to resuscitate a client and prolong life. Kinship laws vary with legal jurisdictions and a next of kin may be able to identify for a client who is unable to make their wishes known what measures should be taken

Advance directives

1. Description
   a. Clients who are competent have the right to complete advance directives for health care which could be followed in the event that they are unable at sometime to make their own decisions.
   b. In many legal jurisdictions, next of kin may request additional medical measures to prolong life.

Issues related to death and dying

1. Description
   a. An older adult may have an advance directive with which family members disagree.
   b. Older adults may delegate important decisions to family members who do not understand the ramifications of health care choices they may make such as putting a client with end stage congestive heart failure on a ventilator.

> **NURSING ALERT**
>
> I t is the duty of the RN to assist family members in understanding complex medical care and to help them formulate questions to ask physicians concerning the quality and quantity of life for the client.

Abuse and neglect of vulnerable older adults
1. Description
    a. Older adults may be the victims of emotional, physical and sexual abuse.
    b. The registered nurse must be alert to the signs of abuse and neglect, possibly from caregivers.
    c. Signs of abuse include unexplained bruises or welts, multiples bruises, unexplained fractures, abrasions, and lacerations, multiple injuries, withdrawal or passivity, fear, depression and hopelessness.
    d. Signs of neglect include dehydration, malnourishment, over medication or under medication, desertion or abandonment, inappropriate or soiled clothes, lack of glasses, dentures or other aides if usually worn, and being left unattended.
    e. Exploitation of the vulnerable older adult includes disappearance of possessions, forced to sell possessions or change a will, overcharged for home repairs, inadequate living environment, inability to afford social activities, being forced to sign over control of finances, and no money for food or clothes.
    f. The registered nurse must report abuse, neglect and exploitation to the proper authorities.

REVIEW QUESTIONS

1. A nurse admitted an older adult with a history of alcohol abuse. The client asked for assurance that leather restraints would not be used under any circumstances during alcohol withdrawal after surgery. The nurse promised that no restraints would be used. After surgery, the client was very agitated, delirious, and combative. Although restraints were indicated to preserve the client's safety, the nurse opposed using them because of the promise made. This action by the nurse was

    1. appropriate because of the nurse's promise.
    2. inappropriate because the promise was not safe.
    3. a violation of the American Nurses Association Code of Ethics for Nurses.
    4. a violation of the American Nurses Association Nursing Standards.

2. A staff member observes a nurse assigned to a postoperative nursing unit reading the chart of a friend's grandmother who is a client on the unit. The nurse is not assigned to this client and does not have a responsibility for this client's care. The client was just diagnosed with terminal cancer and the family does not know. The staff member evaluates the action by the nurse as

   1. appropriate because the nurse is a health care worker and assigned to the unit.
   2. inappropriate because the grandmother is not assigned to the nurse.
   3. not being a violation of the client's privacy because the nurse does not tell anyone what is in the chart.
   4. gaining information to assist a friend through a difficult time.

3. The nurse is concerned about the medical care a long-term care resident is receiving. The nurse asks an opinion about the medical care from a physician who is not responsible for the client. The nurse has

   1. violated the principle of confidentiality.
   2. acted appropriately to gain information on the client's behalf.
   3. gone to the appropriate chain of command.
   4. followed institutional policy.

4. A nursing home resident is offered the opportunity to participate in research on a new drug therapy to treat pressure ulcers. The resident decides after signing the consent form not to participate in the research project. Based on an understanding of the legal issues related to nursing homes, which of the following is appropriate in this situation? The client

   1. cannot withdraw from the study after the consent is signed.
   2. can withdraw at any time from the study.
   3. cannot participate in a study because of being incompetent.
   4. can withdraw only if the family requests withdrawal.

5. The nurse is eating lunch in a nursing home cafeteria. Two nurse aides can be heard at the next table talking about a resident by name. Which of the following is the priority nursing action?

   1. Talk to the nurse aides privately later about this inappropriate behavior
   2. Tell the nurse aides they are being overheard and should talk quietly
   3. Report them to their supervisor
   4. Tell the nurse aides that they are breaching confidentiality

6. The nurse is working in an outpatient same day surgery unit. An 86-year-old client signs the surgical consent form and asks the nurse, "What did I

just sign? My wife always takes care of the paperwork." Which of the following is the priority nursing action?

1. Assess what the client understands about the surgery

2. Notify the surgeon that the client does not understand the surgery

3. Ask the client's wife to explain the consent for surgery

4. Ask the client's wife to sign the consent form because the client is not competent

7. Which of the following is the appropriate nursing action when a nursing student assigned to the surgery suite for observation asks the nurse for permission to photocopy the surgical record from a client's chart for an assignment the student must write?

1. Photocopy the pages for the student

2. Allow the student to photocopy the pages without the client's name

3. Allow the student to write down pertinent but no identifying information

4. Ask the physician for permission to photocopy the pages

8. The nurse working in a long-term care facility is orientating a new nurse to the facility. The nurse should tell the new nurse that which of the following is the priority reason that health care issues of older adults become an ethical dilemma?

1. The choices for health care options do not seem to be clearly right or wrong

2. Decisions are made based on value systems

3. Decisions are made quickly

4. The legal rights of the client coexist with the health professional's obligation to provide care for the client

9. The nurse informs a nursing student that the document that permits an older adult to list the medical treatment refused if unable to make decisions is called _____ .

10. The temporary nurse from a registry is working on the night shift in a long-term care facility. This nurse has had little experience working with the older adult. Which of the following is an appropriate assignment for the charge nurse to give the nurse from the registry?

1. An 83-year-old hospice client who is expected to die soon

2. Administration of medication to 18 clients

3. Six clients who are stable

4. Two clients with fevers of unknown origin

11. The nurse is planning care for a group of older adult clients. Which of the following clients is a priority for the nurse to care for first?

    1. An 87-year-old client in need of a dressing change

    2. An 83-year-old client with an infected total knee replacement incision

    3. A 92-year-old client who has a temperature of 38.3°C, or 101°F

    4. A 90-year-old client who has potassium of 6.7 mEq/L

12. A nurse is teaching a class of new graduate nurses on negligence. Which of the following situations is a priority for the nurse to include in the class as an example of negligence?

    1. Not giving a prescribed medication to an older adult

    2. Not turning off the oxygen at the bedside when a client at home wants to smoke in bed

    3. Not allowing a family member to awaken an older adult client who is sleeping

    4. Talking about a client outside of the long-term care facility

13. One of the unlicensed assistive personnel (UAPs) caring for an older adult with fragile skin report to the nurse a red, painful, and swollen IV site in the hand. Which of the following requests by the nurse does the UAP interpret as inappropriate and illegal?

    1. "Tell the client I'll be there as soon as I can."

    2. "Carefully take the IV out."

    3. "Put a cool washcloth on the IV site."

    4. "Elevate the client's hand on a pillow."

14. After reviewing the records of four older clients in a long-term care facility, which of the following situations does the nurse recognize as violating the client's right to privacy?

    1. Administering a medication to a client in the presence of other clients

    2. Placing the client's name on the client's bed

    3. Placing a photograph of the client in the medication administration record

    4. Placing a photograph of the client in the medical record

15. A 66-year-old client is admitted to a long-term care facility for rehabilitation following a total hip replacement. The client refuses to stay in the facility and tells the nurse, "I am going to walk home." Which of the following is the appropriate action by the nurse?

1. Tell the client that rehabilitation is necessary and leaving is not possible
2. Restrain the client to prevent the client from leaving
3. Call security to restrain the client
4. Do not prohibit the client from leaving

16. The older adult client in a long-term care facility is soiled with feces. The client calls out, "Stop, don't hurt me. Help!" while being bathed by the nurse. Because the nurse did not have the client or the client's guardian's expressed permission to bathe the client, the nurse is at risk for being accused of misconduct results in injury to the client. Negligence is the failure to do something that a reasonable person, led by those ordinary considerations that ordinarily regulate human affairs, would do, or the doing of something another reasonable person would not do.

    1. assault.
    2. battery.
    3. malpractice.
    4. negligence.

17. A 66-year-old client with developmental disabilities and schizophrenia living in a long-term care facility develops pneumonia and is seriously ill. There are no advance directives and no legal guardian. Which of the following is the appropriate nursing intervention as the client's condition worsens?

    1. Do not resuscitate because of the impairment of the client
    2. Do not resuscitate because of the age of the client
    3. Provide all possible medical treatment including resuscitation
    4. Call the client's physician for a do not resuscitate order

18. A nurse observes a staff member telling an older adult client that if the client does not take prescribed oral medications, dessert will be withheld. The nurse reports the behavior of the staff member as

    1. assault.
    2. battery.
    3. malpractice.
    4. negligence.

19. A new employee to a long-term care facility asks the nurse if pictures of the residents may be taken. The appropriate response is, "Pictures

    1. cannot be published without the resident's or guardian's permission."
    2. may only be taken by the family."

3. can be published if the residents are not identified."

4. will not violate the right to privacy when taken discreetly."

20. An older adult client receives a gift of boxed chocolate candy. The client has dementia and does not understand that the candy is the client's and what it is. The nurse should

   1. tell the client the candy is the client's and offer a piece.

   2. offer the candy to the other clients.

   3. send the candy home with the client's family.

   4. throw the candy away, since the client is unable to eat it.

21. Based on an understanding of the legal liability in health care, a nurse who fails to monitor the bowel movement pattern of an older adult client, which leads to an impaction, has committed _____ .

22. A nurse allowed an older adult who is confused to hold onto her purse. Later, the client was receiving oxygen by nasal prongs and attempted to light a cigarette with a cigarette lighter from the purse. An explosion, fire, and injury subsequently resulted. The case goes to court and the nurse is charged with _____ .

23. An older adult client tells the nurse that the client has human immunodeficiency virus (HIV). The nurse should

   1. document this information in the client's chart.

   2. tell the client's physician.

   3. inform the health care team who will come in contact with the client.

   4. encourage the client to disclose this information to the client's physician.

24. The nurse caring for an older adult tears the skin of the client while removing a piece of tape. The skin is attached to the upper arm and to the tape. The nurse cuts the attached part of the skin with a scissors in order to remove the tape. The nurse fails to understand that if harm comes to the client during the act of cutting the skin with the scissors, which of the following could the nurse be charged with?

   1. Malpractice

   2. Negligence

   3. Acceptable practice

   4. Assault

25. The nurse caring for an older adult client soiled with feces fails to clean and bathe the client, leaving the client for another staff member to care for. Another nurse reports this nurse as guilty of

   1. nonmaleficence.

   2. negligence.

3. malpractice.

4. assault.

26. Which of the following should the nurse include when teaching a class on restraint application in the older adult?

   1. Restraints should be removed and reapplied every four hours

   2. Place a client with extremity restraints in a prone position to ensure safety

   3. A physician must evaluate a client within one hour after restraints are applied in an emergency situation

   4. A client should have a belt restraint on at all times as a safety precaution

27. The nurse should include which of the following in the plan of care for a client who is confused, combative, bedridden, and has a vest restraint?

   1. Securely tie the straps of the vest restraint to the side rails of the bed

   2. Crisscross the vest in the front and tie the vest with a quick-release knot

   3. Remove the client's gown before applying the vest to ensure a snug fit

   4. Provide hygienic care around the vest, taking care not to untie or remove the vest

28. The nurse is caring for an older adult client who is very combative and is constantly hitting the staff at a long-term care facility. The decision was made that extremity restraints are temporarily necessary. Which of the following is most appropriate to include in this client's plan of care?

   1. Place the client in a lateral position

   2. Insert one finger between the restraint and the client's extremity

   3. Secure the restraint to the nonmovable part of the bed

   4. Remove the restraint after four hours to assess the skin

29. The nurse appropriately applies a mummy restraint to which of the following clients?

   1. An older adult client who is confused

   2. A screaming child prior to an eye irrigation

   3. An adolescent who is having a drug reaction

   4. An older adult client who is combative and scratching the staff

30. The registered nurse is preparing to delegate nursing tasks. Which of the following should the nurse delegate to unlicensed assistive personnel?

   1. Perform a neurovascular assessment on an older adult client who has a jacket restraint

   2. Assess the skin integrity of an older adult client with a belt restraint

3. Perform range-of-motion exercises on an older adult client with an extremity restraint

4. Assess the oxygenation status of an older adult client with a vest restraint

31. The registered nurse is preparing the client assignments for the day in a long-term care facility. Which of the following client assignments would be appropriate for the registered nurse to delegate to unlicensed personnel?
    1. Application of a prescribed restraint
    2. Administration of medications through a nasogastric tube
    3. Assessment of a postoperative stoma
    4. Irrigation of a Foley catheter

ANSWERS AND RATIONALES

1. 2. The nurse should not have made a promise that would possibly compromise the client's safety. The client could also receive some medication for the agitation, delirium, or combative behavior.

2. 2. Nurses only have the right to health care information that involves the clients for whom they are responsible and to whom the nurses have a duty.

3. 1. A resident of a long-term facility, as other clients, has the right to confidentiality about personal health care information. If the nurse has a concern, the matter should be discussed with the primary physician.

4. 2. Even though living in a long-term care facility, the older adult is considered competent unless legally declared otherwise. A client can withdraw from a research study at any time.

5. 4. Residents of a nursing home, as all clients, have the right to confidentiality. The priority action is to deal with this inappropriate behavior as soon as it occurs. The nurse has the responsibility to protect the resident's privacy.

6. 1. Assessment of the client's understanding of the surgery is essential. If a client has signed a surgical consent form then questions what was signed, it is a priority to assess what the client understands. After assessing what the client understands, or if the client is incompetent, then it would be appropriate to notify the physician.

7. 3. When a nursing student wants to photocopy a client's medical record, nonidentifying information may be written down. The client has the right to confidentiality and any information that could be linked to the client, such as names or addresses, cannot be shared.

8. 4. Although health care options do not seem clearly right or wrong and decisions in a long-term care facility are made quickly, the priority reason health care issues in older adults become highly charged ethical dilemmas is that the client's rights to care and for a dignified death are managed in the context of the health professional's obligations to provide care.

9. **Advance directive.** An advance directive is a document that outlines the medical treatments a person chooses to refuse if unable to make decisions.

10. 3. A nurse who is not familiar with the agency or the clients should be assigned to the most stable clients. Assigning a nurse to a hospice client, to clients with fevers of unknown etiology, or to administering medication to clients all require knowledge of the particular clients.

11. 4. Although a client with an infected knee replacement, a temperature of 38.3°C, or 101°F, and a client in need of a dressing change all need an assessment by the nurse, the client with a potassium level of 6.7 mEq/L is the most acute and at risk.

12. 2. Negligence is the result of either omitting to do something that another reasonable person, guided by those ordinary considerations that ordinarily regulate human affairs, would do, or of doing something another reasonable or prudent person would not do. If there is imminent danger to a client, the nurse must take every measure to protect the client. It may be appropriate for the nurse such as in the case of a client with a sudden rash and the nurse withholds a prescribed antibiotic, which may contribute to the development of the rash. It is inappropriate to talk about a client outside of a long-term care facility because it violates the client's right to privacy, but it is not negligence.

13. 2. Unlicensed assistive personnel cannot legally perform a nursing function such as removing an IV. This would be interpreted as inappropriate and illegal.

14. 1. The medications that a client receives are private. The medications should not be administered where someone else, such as another client, can see what the client is receiving. Placing the client's name on the client's bed, and placing a photograph in the client's medical record or medication administration record are for the client's safety and do not violate the right to privacy. Only authorized personnel have access to that information.

15. 4. A client who is in a long-term care facility for rehabilitation and who wants to go home is competent and able to make decisions, even if those decisions may endanger the client's health. It would be inappropriate to prevent the client from leaving, because the client can make health care decisions unless incompetence has been declared. Restraining the client would be false imprisonment or battery.

16. **2.** Because the client is protesting the bathing, the nurse could be accused of battery without the permission of the guardian. Battery is the unlawful touching of another person. Assault is an unjustifiable attempt or a threat to touch a person without consent that results in fear of immediate harm. The touching may not actually occur. Malpractice is a type of negligence in which any unreasonable act or professional misconduct results in injury to the client. Negligence is the failure to do something that a reasonable person, led by those ordinary considerations that ordinarily regulate human affairs, would do, or the doing of something another reasonable person would not do.

17. **3.** In the absence of advance directives by the client or a guardian, the nurse must provide all appropriate care.

18. **1.** Assault is a deliberate threat that the client believes could be carried through, or an unjustifiable attempt or threat to touch a person without consent that results in fear of immediate harm. Battery is unlawful touching of another person. Malpractice is a type of negligence in which any unreasonable act or professional misconduct results in injury to the client. Negligence is the omission of doing something that a reasonable person, led by those ordinary considerations that ordinarily regulate human affairs, would do or doing something another reasonable person would not do.

19. **1.** The right to privacy includes the publishing of pictures or any other information about a client without the client's or guardian's permission. The nurse has the responsibility to advocate for and protect the client's privacy. Pictures may be taken in a long-term care facility for the purpose of placing the photograph in the client's medical record or on the medication administration record.

20. **1.** When a client with dementia does not recognize that candy gift belongs to the client, the nurse should take every opportunity to get the client to enjoy it. The candy is a gift and the personal property of the client. The nurse cannot take the candy. This could constitute larceny.

21. **Negligence.** Negligence is the omission or commission of an act that departs from the acceptable and reasonable standards of practice. The nurse is expected to monitor the elimination patterns of clients.

22. **Criminal negligence.** Criminal negligence is the disregard of protecting the safety of another person. The nurse has the responsibility to protect the client. In this case, the nurse failed to protect the client with oxygen from lighting cigarettes with a lighter and sustaining injury.

23. **4.** The nurse must protect the client's right to privacy of health care information. Documenting a client's HIV status in the client's chart, telling the client's physician, and informing the health care team who will come in contact with the client all violate the client's right to privacy.

24. 1. Cutting the skin of a client with a scissors could be considered a medical procedure and not within the scope of nursing practice. A charge of malpractice could result. Malpractice is a type of negligence in which any unreasonable act or professional misconduct results in injury to the client. Negligence is the omission or commission of an act that departs from the acceptable and reasonable standards of practice. Assault is an unjustifiable attempt or threat to touch a person without consent that results in fear of immediate harm. The touching may not actually occur.

25. 2. The nurse is failing to perform an expected action, keeping the client clean and safe from harm. This is negligence. Negligence is the omission or commission of an act that departs from the acceptable and reasonable standards of practice. Malpractice is a type of negligence in which any unreasonable act or professional misconduct results in injury to the client. Assault is an unjustifiable attempt or threat to touch a person without consent that results in fear of immediate harm. The touching may not actually occur. Nonmaleficence is a principle that requires the nurse to act in such a way as to prevent harm to a client.

26. 3. The least restrictive type of restraint should be used. If restraints are used in an emergency situation, a physician must evaluate the client within one hour after the restraint is applied. Restraints should be reassessed every hour and removed every two hours. Wrist and ankle restraints should not be applied with the client in a prone position because there is an increased risk for aspiration. The client should be placed in a supine position. A belt restraint should not be used just because the client is an older adult and without justification. This is considered false imprisonment.

27. 2. A vest restraint should be crisscrossed in the front and tied with a quick-release knot. The restraint should be applied over the client's clothes to prevent friction on the skin. A restraint should never be tied to the side rails of the bed. This poses the risk of strangulation.

28. 1. A client who has an extremity restraint should be placed in the lateral position. Placing this client in a supine position would place the client at risk for aspiration. Two fingers should be inserted under a restraint to prevent it from being too tight. The restraint should never be applied to the nonmovable part of the bed, to avoid the restraint from becoming too tight when the bed is raised or lowered. The skin under a restraint must be assessed every hour and the restraint must be removed every two hours.

29. 2. A mummy restraint is most generally used with a small child during some kind of short-term examination or treatment. Older adult clients

should never be restrained because they are confused or combative. An adolescent would never be restrained just because of a drug reaction.

30. 3. Performing specific assessments, such as a neurovascular or an oxygenation assessment, or checking for skin integrity should not be delegated to unlicensed assistive personnel. These tasks require the skills of a nurse. Unlicensed assistive personnel may perform range-of-motion exercises on a client who has a restraint.

31. 1. Although unlicensed assistive personnel should not perform any assessments on a client with a restraint, they have been trained to apply the restraint. Administration of medications through a nasogastric tube, assessment of a postoperative stoma, and irrigation of a Foley catheter should be performed by a nurse.

Appendices Table of Contents

Appendix A: Application of Cultural Phenomena to Nursing Care

Cultural Group	Communication	Space	Time Orientation	Social Organization	Environmental Control	Biological Variations	Nursing Implications
African American	Language(s): • English Silence: • Head-nodding does not mean agreement. Eye contact: • Direct eye contact is often viewed as being rude. Other: • Nonverbal communication is very important. • It is intrusive to ask personal questions of someone one has just met.	Social distance: • Close, personal space Touch: • Touching anothers hair is sometimes viewed as offensive.	• Present over future • Flexible concept of time	Family: • Large, extended family networks are important. Gender roles: • Women serve as both bread winners and caretakers. Religion: • Protestant (Baptist) • Strong church affiliation with community Other: • Social organizations are strong within communities	Definition of health: • Harmony with nature • No separation of body, mind, and spirit Causative factors of illness: • Disharmonious state that may be caused by demons or spirits • Can be prevented by nutritious meals, rest, and cleanliness	Dietary practices and preferences: • Foods are slow-cooked in added fat • Some pregnant African Americans engage in pica (ingestion of nonfood items, such as laundry starch). Increased susceptibility: • Lactose intolerance • Keloid formation • Sickle cell anemia • Hypertension • Cancer (especially stomach and esophageal) • Coronary heart disease	• Encourage involvement of extended family. • Know that a folk healer (or herbalist) may be consulted before individual seeks other treatment. • Clarify meaning and intent of client's words. • Validate the meaning of client's nonverbal behavior. • Avoid rigidly scheduling care procedures; be flexible with use of time.

Asian American	Language(s):	Social distance:	Present	Family:	Definition of health:	Dietary practices and preferences:	

	• Chinese (especially Mandarin)
	• Japanese
	• Korean
	• Vietnamese
	• English
	
	Silence:
	• Is valued
	
	Eye contact:
	• Considered to be rude
	
	Other:
	• Criticism or disagreement is not expressed verbally.
	• The word no is avoided to show respect for others.
	• An up-turned palm is offensive.
		• Avoid physical closeness
		
		Touch:
		• Usually do not touch others during conversation
		• Is unacceptable with members of opposite sex
		
		Touch:
		• Touching someone on the head is disrespectful because the head is considered to be sacred.
				• Highly value immediate and extended family
				• Honor elders and ancestors
				• Family unit is very structured and hierarchical.
				• Family loyalty and honor are valued.
				
				Gender roles:
				• Men have the power and authority.
				• Women are expected to be obedient.
				
				Religion:
				• Taoism
				• Buddhism
				• Islam
				• Christianity
				
				Other:
				• Education is viewed as important.
					• A state of physical and spiritual harmony with nature
					• A balance between positive and negative energy forces (yin and yang)
					• A healthy body is viewed as a gift from ancestors.
					
					Causative factors of illness:
					• Yin and yang imbalance
					• Contributing factors include:
					  –Prolonged sitting or lying
					  –Overexertion
						• Soy sauce
						• Raw fish
						• Rice
						
						Increased susceptibility:
						• Lactose intolerance
						• Hypertension
						• Cancer (stomach and liver)
							• Expect that a traditional healer will probably be consulted first.
							• Clarify responses to questions.
							• Avoid excessive touch.
							• Limit eye contact.
							• Avoid gesturing with your hands.
							• Only touch the client's head when necessary and explain before doing so.
							• Avoid rigidly scheduling care procedures; be flexible with time use.

Continued

Cultural Group	Communication	Space	Time Orientation	Social Organization	Environmental Control	Biological Variations	Nursing Implications
European American	Language(s): • National languages • English Silence: • Can be used to show respect or disdain for another, depending on the situation Eye contact: • Indicates trust-worthiness	Social distance: • Tend to avoid close physical contact • Aloof Touch: • Handshakes for formal greetings	• Future over present	Family: • Nuclear family is basic unit. • Extended family is important. Gender roles: • The male is the dominant figure. Religion: • Judeo-Christian Other: • Community social organizations are important.	Definition of health: • Usually viewed as absence of disease or illness Causative factors of illness: • Often viewed as punishment for sins • Tend to be stoical when expressing complaints	Dietary practices and preferences: • Carbohydrates (potatoes) • Red meat Increased susceptibility: • Heart disease • Thalassemia • Breast cancer • Diabetes	• Focus on client's body language. • Respect client's personal space. • Help client decrease fatalistic viewpoint of illness. • Know that home remedies may be the first method of treatment used.
Hispanic American	Language(s): • Spanish or Portuguese with many dialects Silence: • Tend to be verbally expressive	Social distance: • Comfortable with close proximity to others Touch: • Very tactile (use of embraces, handshakes)	• Present oriented • Concept of time is flexible.	Family: • Nuclear family is basic unit. • Extended family is highly regarded. • Needs of family take precedence	Definition of health: • May be a reward from God or the result of good luck • Results from a state of balance between "hot" and "cold" forces and	Dietary practices and preferences: • Beans • Fried foods • Spicy foods Increased susceptibility: • Lactose intolerance	• Offer to call priest or other clergy because of significance of religious practices related to illness (e.g., sacrament of anointing the sick person).

Eye contact:
- Eye behavior is significant. The "evil eye" can be given to a child if a person looks at and admires a child without touching the child.
- Avoidance of eye contact indicates respect and attentiveness.

Other:
- Direct confrontation is disrespectful.
- Dramatic body language (gestures, facial expressions) is used to express emotions or pain.
- Confidentiality is important.
- Expression of negative feelings is impolite.

- Values physical presence of others

Other:
- Politeness is essential.
- Modesty is necessary.

over needs of individual.

Gender roles:
- Man is the decision maker and breadwinner.
- Woman is care-taker and homemaker.

Religion:
- Catholicism

"wet" and "dry" forces

Causative factors of illness:
- God's punishment for sins
- *Susto* (fright)
- *Mal ojo* (evil eye)
- *Envidia* (envy)

- Diabetes
- Parasites

- Protect privacy.
- Maintain confidentiality.
- Communicate with male head of family.
- Always touch a child you are admiring or examining.
- Avoid rigidly scheduling care procedures; be flexible with use of time.
- Pay particular attention to dietary preferences.

Continued

Cultural Group	Communication	Space	Time Orientation	Social Organization	Environmental Control	Biological Variations	Nursing Implications
Native American (Referred to as Native American in the United States and as Aboriginals in Canada)	Language(s): • English • Tribal languages Silence: • Indicates respect for the speaker Eye contact: • Is avoided because it is a sign of disrespect Other: • Body language is important mode of communication • Speak in low tone of voice. • Expect others to be attentive.	Social distance: • Personal space is very important. • Space has no boundaries. Touch: • Will lightly touch another person's hand during greetings • Massages given to newborns to promote bonding between infant and mother. • Touching a dead body is prohibited.	• Usually present oriented	Family: • Basic unit is extended family, often including people from several households. • Very family-oriented • In some tribes, grandparents are viewed as family leaders. • Elders are honored. Gender roles: • The father does all the work outside the home. • The mother assumes responsibility for domestic duties.	Definition of health: • Health is a state of harmony between the person, the family, and the environment. Causative factors of illness: • Supernatural forces • Disequilibrium between person and environment • Everything that happens is the result of something else (past or future events)	Dietary practices and preferences: • Vary greatly according to tribal customs and geographical location. • Navajos prefer meat and blue cornmeal and tend to avoid the consumption of milk. Increased susceptibility: • Tuberculosis • Diabetes • Heart disease • Arthritis • American Eskimos are susceptible to glaucoma. • Because there are over 400	• Elicit input from extended family members. • Actively accommodate extended family visitors in hospital and clinic settings. • In the home, modify infection control and hygiene practices according to availability of resources. • Closely monitor own use of body language. • Encourage client to personalize space in which health care is delivered (e.g.,

Religion:

- Sacred myths and legends provide spiritual guidance.
- Religion and healing practices are blended with each other.

Other:

- Community social organizations are important.
- Children are taught to respect traditions.

tribes in North America (including Eskimos and Aleuts), expect diversity according to specific tribe.

bring personal items, objects to hospital room).
- Clarify messages.
- Understand that the client may be attentive even when eye contact is absent.

SOURCE: *Date adapted from Spector, R. E. (2004). Cultural diversity in health and illness (6th ed.). Upper Saddle River, NJ: Prentice-Hall. Stanhope, M., & Lancaster, J. (2004). Community and public health nursing (6th ed.). St. Louis, MO: Mosby.*

Appendix B: Nursing Checklist for Culturally Sensitive Care

1. Assess and incorporate family history of health care:
   - Fluency in English
   - Extent of family support or disintegration of family
   - Community resources
   - Level of education
   - Change of social status as a result of coming to this country
   - Intimate relationships with people of different backgrounds
   - Level of stress
2. Affirm client strengths and potential for growth.
3. Recognize informal caregivers (family members and significant others) as an integral part of treatment.
4. Demonstrate caring behaviors rather than just tolerating cultural variations in client's behavior.

Appendix C: Cultural Assessment Interview Guide

Cultural Assessment Interview Guide

Name: _____

Nickname or other names or special meaning attributed to your name: _____

Primary language:

      When speaking _____

      When writing _____

Date of birth: _____

Place of birth: _____

Educational level or specialized training: _____

To which ethnic group do you belong? _____

To what extent do you identify with your cultural group? _____

Who is the spokesperson for your family? _____

Describe some of the customs or beliefs that you have about the following:

      Health _____

      Life _____

      Illness _____

      Death _____

How do you learn information best?

    ☐ Reading

    ☐ Having someone explain verbally

    ☐ Having someone demonstrate

Describe some of your family's dietary habits and your personal food preferences. _____

_____

Are there any foods forbidden from your diet for religious or cultural reasons? _____

_____

Describe your religious affiliation. _____

What role do your religious beliefs and practices play in your life during times of good health and bad health? _____

_____

Whom do you rely on for health care services or healing and what type of cultural health practices have you been exposed to? _____

_____

Are there any sanctions or restrictions in your culture that the person taking care of you should know? _____

_____

Describe your current living arrangements. _____

How do members of your family communicate with each other? _____

Describe your strengths. _____

Who /what is your primary source of information about your health? _____

Is there anything else that is important about your cultural beliefs that you want to tell me? _____

FIGURE C-1

Appendix D: Leadership Stages

Style	Description	Leader Behaviors	Potential Impact on Group Members	Advantages	Disadvantages
Autocratic	• Basic premise: Leader knows best. • Communication flows downward.	• Controlling • Directive • Makes all decisions and solves all problems • Issues commands	• Hostility • Rebellion	• Task-oriented, high productivity • Facilitates a quick response • Often necessary in crisis situation	• Inhibits creativity and autonomy of members • Promotes mistrust and fear among followers • Members may become hostile or passive
Democratic ("participative leadership")	• Basic premise: Every member should have input. • Communication is open and mutual.	• Acts as a facilitator • Serves as resource person • Encourages members' active participation	• Improved productivity • More opportunity for personal growth • Increased cooperation and teamwork	• Promotes empowerment of team members • Facilitates communication • Increased creativity and autonomy	• Time-consuming • May be less efficient (in quantifiable terms) • Disagreements may happen as members express their viewpoints

| Laissez-faire | • Leadership responsibilities are assumed by group.
• Almost any behavior by the group is permissible due to the leader's lack of limit-setting and stated expectations. | • Passive, nondirective approach
• Provides little, if any, support, guidance, or feedback
• Sets no limits | • Unmet tasks
• Relationship needs of group members ignored
• Apathy | • Promotes autonomy and creativity in members | • May evoke passivity in team members.
• Aimless behavior often occurs
• Chaos common
• Inefficiency and low productivity |

Appendix E: Management Theories

Management Theory	Main Contributors	Key Aspects
Scientific management	Frederick Taylor (1856-1915) Frank Gilbreth (1868-1924) Lillian Gilbreth (1878-1972)	Machinelike focus Analysis of elements of an operation Training of the worker Use of proper tools and equipment Use of incentives Use of time and motion studies to make the work easier
Bureaucratic theory	Max Weber (1864-1920): German sociologist	Division of labor, hierarchy of authority, and chain of command Rationality, impersonal management Use of merit and skill as basis for promotion/ reward Use of rules and regulations, focus on exacting work processes Career service, salaried managers

Administrative principles	Mary Parker Follet (1868-1933): Trained in philosophy/political science at Radcliffe	The science of management Principles of organization applicable in any setting
	Henri Fayol (1841-1925): French mining engineer, head of major mining company	Fayol's principles: unity of command, division of work, unity of direction, scalar chain, and management functions— planning, organizing, coordinating, and controlling
	Chester Barnard (1886-1961): Harvard economics, president of New Jersey Bell Telephone	Concerned with the optimal approach for administrators to achieve economic efficiency
	Luther Gulick and Lyndal Urwick (1937): *Papers on the Science of Administration*	Planning, organizing, supervising, directing, controlling, organizing, reviewing, and budgeting = POSDCORB
	James Mooney (1939): *Principles of Organization*	Four principles: coordination, hierarchical structure (scalar), functional (division of labor), staff/line principle
Human relations (replaced later with the term *organizational behavior*)	Elton Mayo (1933) Fritz Roethlisberger (1939): Harvard University	Hawthorne studies led to the belief that human relations between workers and managers and among workers were main determinants of efficiency. The Hawthorne effect refers to change in behavior as a result of being watched.

Appendix F: Ethical Principles and Rules

Ethical Principle/ Rule	Definition	Example
Beneficence	The duty to do good to others and to maintain a balance between benefits and harms.	• Provide all patients, including the terminally ill, with caring attention. • Become familiar with your state laws regarding organ donations. • Treat every patient with respect and courtesy.
Nonmaleficence	The principle of doing no harm.	• Always work within your scope of practice. • Never give information or perform duties you are not qualified to do. • Observe all safety rules and precautions. • Keep areas safe from hazards. • Perform procedures according to facility protocols. Never take shortcuts. • Ask an appropriate person about anything you are unsure of. • Keep your skills up to date.

Justice	The principle of fairness that is served when an individual is given that which he or she is due, owed, deserves, or can legitimately claim.	• Treat all patients equally, regardless of economic or social background. • Learn the state laws and your facility's policies and procedures for handling and reporting suspected abuse.
Autonomy	Respect for an individual's right to self-determination; respect for individual liberty.	• Be sure that patients have consented to all treatments and procedures. • Become familiar with state laws and facility policies dealing with advance directives. • Never release patient information of any kind unless there is a signed release. • Do not discuss patients with anyone who is not professionally involved in their care. • Protect the physical privacy of patients.
Fidelity	The principle of promise keeping; the duty to keep one's promise or word.	• Be sure that necessary contracts have been completed. • Be very careful about what you say to patients. They may only hear the "good news."
Respect for others	The right of people to make their own decision.	• Provide all persons with information for decision making. • Avoid making paternalistic decisions for others.
Veracity	The obligation to tell the truth.	• Admit mistakes promptly. Offer to do whatever is necessary to correct them. • Refuse to participate in any form of fraud. • Give an "honest day's work" every day.

Appendix G: NANDA Nursing Diagnoses 2005–2006

Activity Intolerance

Risk for Activity Intolerance

Impaired Adjustment

Ineffective Airway Clearance

Latex Allergy Response

Risk for Latex Allergy Response

Anxiety

Death Anxiety

Risk for Aspiration

Risk for Impaired Parent/Infant/Child Attachment

Autonomic Dysreflexia

Risk for Autonomic Dysreflexia

Disturbed Body Image

Risk for Imbalanced Body Temperature

Bowel Incontinence

Effective Breastfeeding

Ineffective Breastfeeding

Interrupted Breastfeeding

Ineffective Breathing Pattern

Decreased Cardiac Output

Caregiver Role Strain

Risk for Caregiver Role Strain

Impaired Verbal Communication

Readiness for Enhanced Communication

Decisional Conflict (Specify)

Parental Role Conflict

Acute Confusion

Chronic Confusion

Constipation

Perceived Constipation

Risk for Constipation

Defensive Coping

Ineffective Coping

Readiness for Enhanced Coping

Ineffective Community Coping

Readiness for Enhanced Community Coping

Compromised Family Coping

Disabled Family Coping

Readiness for Enhanced Family Coping

Risk for Sudden Infant Death Syndrome

Ineffective Denial

Impaired Dentition

Risk for Delayed **D**evelopment

Diarrhea

Risk for **D**isuse Syndrome

Deficient **D**iversional Activity

Energy Field Disturbance

Impaired **E**nvironmental Interpretation Syndrome

Adult **F**ailure to Thrive

Risk for **F**alls

Dysfunctional **F**amily Processes: Alcoholism

Interrupted **F**amily Processes

Readiness for Enhanced **F**amily Processes

Fatigue

Fear

Readiness for Enhanced **F**luid Balance

Deficient **F**luid Volume

Excess **F**luid Volume

Risk for Deficient **F**luid Volume

Risk for Imbalanced **F**luid Volume

Impaired **G**as Exchange

Anticipatory **G**rieving

Dysfunctional **G**rieving

Risk for Dysfunctional **G**rieving

Delayed **G**rowth and Development

Risk for Disproportionate **G**rowth

Ineffective **H**ealth Maintenance

Health-Seeking Behaviors (Specify)

Impaired **H**ome Maintenance

Hopelessness

Hyperthermia

Hypothermia

Disturbed Personal **I**dentity

Functional Urinary **I**ncontinence

Reflex Urinary **I**ncontinence

Stress Urinary **I**ncontinence

Total Urinary **I**ncontinence

Urge Urinary **I**ncontinence

Risk for Urge Urinary **I**ncontinence

Disorganized **I**nfant Behavior

Risk for Disorganized **I**nfant Behavior

Readiness for Enhanced Organized **I**nfant Behavior

Ineffective **I**nfant Feeding Pattern

Risk for **I**nfection

Risk for **I**njury

Risk for Perioperative-Positioning **I**njury

Decreased **I**ntracranial Adaptive Capacity

Deficient **K**nowledge

Readiness for Enhanced **K**nowledge (Specify)

Risk for **L**oneliness

Impaired **M**emory

Impaired Bed **M**obility

Impaired Physical **M**obility

Impaired Wheelchair **M**obility

Nausea

Unilateral **N**eglect

Noncompliance

Imbalanced **N**utrition: Less than Body Requirements

Imbalanced **N**utrition: More than Body Requirements

Readiness for Enhanced **N**utrition

Risk for Imbalanced **N**utrition: More than Body Requirements

Impaired **O**ral Mucous Membrane

Acute **P**ain

Chronic **P**ain

Readiness for Enhanced **P**arenting

Impaired Parenting

Risk for Impaired Parenting

Risk for Peripheral Neurovascular Dysfunction

Risk for Poisoning

Post-Trauma Syndrome

Risk for Post-Trauma Syndrome

Powerlessness

Risk for Powerlessness

Ineffective Protection

Rape-Trauma Syndrome

Rape-Trauma Syndrome: Compound Reaction

Rape-Trauma Syndrome: Silent Reaction

Impaired Religiosity

Readiness for Enhanced Religiosity

Risk for Impaired Religiosity

Relocation Stress Syndrome

Risk for Relocation Stress Syndrome

Ineffective Role Performance

Sedentary Life Style

Bathing/Hygiene Self-Care Deficit

Dressing/Grooming Self-Care Deficit

Feeding Self-Care Deficit

Toileting Self-Care Deficit

Readiness for Enhanced Self-Concept

Chronic Low Self-Esteem

Situational Low Self-Esteem

Risk for Situational Low Self-Esteem

Self-Mutilation

Risk for Self-Mutilation

Disturbed Sensory Perception (Specify: Visual, Auditory, Kinesthetic, Gustatory, Tactile, Olfactory)

Sexual Dysfunction

Ineffective Sexuality Patterns

Impaired Skin Integrity

Risk for Impaired Skin Integrity

Sleep Deprivation

Disturbed Sleep Pattern

Readiness for Enhanced Sleep

Impaired Social Interaction

Social Isolation

Chronic Sorrow

Spiritual Distress

Risk for Spiritual Distress

Readiness for Enhanced Spiritual Well-Being

Risk for Suffocation

Risk for Suicide

Delayed Surgical Recovery

Impaired Swallowing

Effective Therapeutic Regimen Management

Ineffective Therapeutic Regimen Management

Readiness for Enhanced Management of Therapeutic Regimen

Ineffective Community Therapeutic Regimen Management

Ineffective Family Therapeutic Regimen Management

Ineffective Thermoregulation

Disturbed Thought Processes

Impaired Tissue Integrity

Ineffective Tissue Perfusion (Specify Type: Renal, Cerebral, Cardiopulmonary, Gastrointestinal, Peripheral)

Impaired Transfer Ability

Risk for Trauma

Impaired Urinary Elimination

Readiness for Enhanced Urinary
Elimination

Urinary Retention

Impaired Spontaneous
Ventilation

Dysfunctional Ventilatory Weaning
Response

Risk for Other-Directed Violence

Risk for Self-Directed Violence

Impaired Walking

Wandering

Appendix H: Preparation for NCLEX

A new graduate from an educational program that prepares registered nurses will take the NCLEX, the national nursing licensure examination prepared under the supervision of the National Council of State Boards of Nursing. NCLEX is taken after graduation and prior to practice as a registered nurse. The examination is given across the United States. Graduates submit their credentials to the state board of nursing in the state in which licensure is desired. Once the state board accepts the graduate's credentials, the graduate can schedule the examination. This examination ensures a basic level of safe registered nursing practice to the public. The examination follows a test plan formulated on four categories of client needs that registered nurses commonly encounter. The concepts of the nursing process, caring, communication, cultural awareness, documentation, self-care, and teaching/learning are integrated throughout the four major categories of client needs (Table H-1).

■ TOTAL NUMBER OF QUESTIONS ON NCLEX

Graduates may receive anywhere from 75 to 265 questions on the NCLEX examination during their testing session. Fifteen of the questions are questions that are being piloted to determine their validity for use in future NCLEX examinations. Students cannot determine whether they passed or failed the NCLEX examination from the number of questions they receive during their session. There is no time limit for each question, and the maximum time for the examination is 5 hours. A 10-minute break is mandatory after 2 hours of testing. An optional 10-minute break may be taken after another 90 minutes of testing.

Each test question has a test item and four possible answers. If the student answers the question correctly, a slightly more difficult item will follow, and the level of difficulty will increase with each item until the candidate misses an item. If the student misses an item, a slightly less difficult item will follow, and the level of difficulty will decrease with each item until the student has answered an item correctly. This process continues until the student has

TABLE H-1   NCLEX Test Plan: Client Needs

Client Needs Tested	Percent of Test Questions
Safe, effective care environment:	
Management of care	7–13%
Safety and infection control	5–11%
Physiologic integrity:	
Basic care and comfort	7–13%
Pharmacological and parenteral therapies	5–11%
Reduction of risk potential	12–18%
Physiological adaptation	12–18%
Psychosocial integrity:	
Coping and adaptation	5–11%
Psychosocial adaptation	5–11%
Health promotion and maintenance:	
Growth and development through the life span	7–13%
Prevention and early detection of disease	5–11%

achieved a definite passing or definite failing score. The least number of questions a student can take to complete the exam is 75. Fifteen of these questions will be pilot questions, and they will not count toward the student's score. The other 60 questions will determine the student's score on the NCLEX.

■ RISK FACTORS FOR NCLEX PERFORMANCE

Several factors have been identified as being associated with performance on the NCLEX examination. Some of these factors are identified in Table H-2.

■ REVIEW BOOKS AND COURSES

In preparing to take the NCLEX, the new graduate may find it useful to review several of the many NCLEX review books on the market. These review books often include a review of nursing content, or sample test questions, or both. They frequently include computer software disks with test questions for review. The test questions may be arranged in the review book by clinical content area, or they may be presented in one or more comprehensive examinations covering all areas of the NCLEX. Listings of these review books are available at *www.amazon.com*. It is helpful to use several of these books and computer software when reviewing for the NCLEX.

TABLE H-2   Factors Associated with NCLEX Performance

- HESI Exit Exam
- Mosby Assesstest
- NLN Comprehensive Achievement test
- NLN achievement tests taken at end of each nursing course
- Verbal SAT score
- ACT score
- High school rank and GPA
- Undergraduate nursing program GPA
- GPA in science and nursing theory courses
- Competency in American English language
- Reasonable family responsibilities or demands
- Absence of emotional distress
- Critical thinking competency

NCLEX review courses are also available. Brochures advertising these programs are often sent to schools and are available in many sites nationwide. The quality of these programs can vary, and students may want to ask former nursing graduates and faculty for recommendations.

■ THE NLN EXAMINATION AND THE HESI EXIT EXAM

Many nursing programs administer an examination to students at the completion of their nursing program. Two of these exams are the NLN Achievement test and the HESI Exit Exam. New graduates will want to review their performance on any of these exams because these results will help identify their weaknesses and help focus their review sessions.

Students who examine their feedback from the NLN examination or the HESI Exit Exam have important information that can help them focus their review for the NCLEX. A strategy for examining this feedback and organizing this review is outlined in the following section.

■ ORGANIZING YOUR REVIEW

In preparing for NCLEX, identify your strengths and weaknesses. If you have taken the NLN examination or the HESI Exit Exam, note any content strength and weakness areas. Additionally, note any nursing program course or clinical content areas in which you scored below a grade of B. Purchase one or more of the NCLEX review books. It is useful to review questions developed by different authors. Review content in the review books in any of your weak content areas. Take a comprehensive exam in the review book or on the computer software disk and analyze your performance. Try to answer as many questions correctly as you can. Be sure to actually practice taking the examinations. Do not just jump ahead to look at the section on correct answers and rationales before answering the questions if you want to improve your examination performance.

TABLE H-3   Preparation for the NCLEX Test

Name: _____

Strengths: _____

Weak content areas identified on NLN examination or HESI Exit Exam:
_____
_____
_____

Weak content areas identified by yourself or others during formal nursing education pro-gram (include content areas in which you scored below a grade of B in class or any factors from Table H-2):
_____
_____
_____

Weak content areas identified in any area of the NCLEX test plan, including the following:
Safe, effective care environment

Physiological integrity

Psychosocial integrity

Health promotion and maintenance

Weak content areas identified in any of the top 10 patient diagnoses in each of the following:
Adult health

Women's health

Mental health nursing

Children's health
   (Consider the 10 top medications, diagnostic tools and tests, treatments and procedures used for each of the ten diagnoses.)

Weak content areas identified in the following:
Therapeutic communication tools

Defense mechanisms

Growth and development

Other

TABLE H-4 Organizing Your NCLEX Study

Note your weaknesses identified in Table H-3.

Take a comprehensive exam from one of the review books and analyze your performance. Then, depending on this test performance and the weaknesses identified in Table H-3, your schedule could look like the following:

Day 1: Practice adult health test questions. Score the test, analyze your performance, and review test question rationales and content weaknesses.

Day 2: Practice women's health test questions. Repeat above process.

Day 3: Practice children's health test questions. Repeat above process.

Day 4: Practice mental health test questions. Repeat above process.

Day 5: Continue with other weak content areas. Continue this process until you are doing well in all areas of the test.

Next, once you have completed the comprehensive examination, review the answers and rationales for any weak content areas and take another comprehensive exam. Repeat this process until you are doing well in all clinical content areas and in all areas of the NCLEX examination plan.

Finally, do a general review of the top 10 patient diseases, medications, diagnostic tests, and nursing procedures in each major nursing content area, as well as defense mechanisms, communication tips, and growth and development. Practice visualization and relaxation techniques as needed. These strategies will assist you in conquering the three areas necessary for successful test taking—anxiety control, content review, and test question practice. Table H-3 will help organize your study.

■ WHEN TO STUDY

Identify your personal best time. Are you a day person? Are you a night person? Study when you are fresh. Arrange to study 1 or more hours daily. Use Table H-4 to organize your study if you have 1 month to go.

Students who use this technique should increase their confidence in their ability to do well on the NCLEX.

Appendix I: Abbreviations

AACN	American Association of Critical-Care Nurses
AACN	American Association of Colleges of Nursing
AAHP	American Association of Health Plans
AAN	American Academy of Nursing
AANA	American Association of Nurse Anesthetists
AARP	American Association of Retired Persons
ACLS	advanced cardiac life support
ACNP	acute care nurse practitioner
ACS	American Cancer Society
ADA	American Dietetic Association
ADL	activity of daily living
ADN	associate degree in nursing
AHA	American Hospital Association
AHRQ	Agency for Healthcare Research and Quality
AIDS	Acquired Immune Deficiency Syndrome
AMA	American Medical Association
ANA	American Nurses Association
ANCC	American Nurses Credentialing Center
AONE	American Organization of Nurse Executives
APC	Ambulatory Payment Classification
APHA	American Public Health Association
AWHONN	Association of Women's Health, Obstetric, and Neonatal Nurses
BLS	basic life support
BMI	body mass index
BSN	bachelor of science in nursing
BTIPA	Brooks' Theory of Intrapersonal Awareness
CAMH	Comprehensive Accreditation Manual for Hospitals
CARING	Capital Area Roundtable on Informatics in Nursing
CCQHC	Consumer Coalition for Quality Health Care
CCRN	critical care registered nurse
CCU	coronary care unit

CDC	Centers for Disease Control and Prevention
CEO	chief executive officer
CEU	continuing education unit
CFO	chief financial officer
CHF	congestive heart failure
CINAHL	Cumulative Index to Nursing and Allied Health Literature
CIS	clinical information system
CMP	comprehensive metabolic panel
CMS	Centers for Medicare and Medicaid Services
CN3	clinical nurse 3
CNA	Canadian Nurses Association
CNM	certified nurse-midwife
CNS	clinical nurse specialist
CNS/NP	clinical nurse specialist/nurse practitioner
CON	certificate of need
COPC	community-oriented primary care
CPR	cardiopulmonary resuscitation
CPR	computerized patient record
CPRI	Computer-based Patient Record Institute
CQI	continuous quality improvement
CRNA	certified registered nurse anesthetist
CU	Consumers Union
CVA	cerebrovascular accident
DM	disease management
DRG	diagnosis-related group
EBC	evidence-based care
EBM	evidence-based medicine
EBNP	evidence-based nursing practice
EBP	evidence-based practice
EMTALA	Emergency Medical Treatment and Active Labor Act
ENIAC	Electronic Numerical Integrator and Computer
ERCP	endoscopic retrograde cholangiopancreatography
ERG	Existence-relatedness-growth theory (Alderfer, 1969)
ET nurse	enterostomal therapy nurse
FTE	full-time equivalent
GI lab	gastrointestinal laboratory
HCFA	Health Care Financing Administration
HIMSS	Health Information and Management Systems Society
HIPAA	Health Insurance Portability and Accountability Act
HIV	human immunodeficiency virus
HMO	health maintenance organization
IADL	instrumental activity of daily living
ICN	International Council of Nurses
ICU	intensive care unit
IOM	Institute of Medicine

IRA	individual retirement account
JBIEBNM	Joanna Briggs Institute for Evidence Based Nursing & Midwifery
JCAHO	Joint Commission on Accreditation of Healthcare Organizations
LOS	length of stay
LPN/LVN	licensed practical nurse/licensed vocational nurse
MBNQA	Malcolm Baldridge National Quality Award
MBTI	Myers-Briggs Type Indicator
MDI	metered-dose inhaler
MEDLARS	Medical Literature Analysis and Retrieval System
MeSH	Medical Subject Headings
MIS	medical information system
MRI	Medical Records Institute
MS-HUG	Microsoft Healthcare Users Group
MSN	master's degree in nursing
NANDA	North American Nursing Diagnosis Association
NANN	National Association of Neonatal Nurses
NAPNAP	National Association of Pediatric Nurses and Practitioners
NAPQ	Nosek-Androwich Profit: Quality Matrix
NCLEX	National Council Licensure Examination
NCQA	National Committee on Quality Assurance
NCSBN	National Council of State Boards of Nursing
NGC	National Guideline Clearinghouse
NHPPD	nursing hours per patient day
NIH	National Institutes of Health
NLM	National Library of Medicine
NLN	National League for Nursing
NNP	neonatal nurse practitioner
NP	nurse practitioner
NRP	neonatal resuscitation program
NWIG-AMIA	Nursing Working Informatics Group of the American Medical Informatics Association
OR	operating room
OSHA	Occupational Safety and Health Administration
PALS	pediatric advanced life support
PC	personal computer
PCA	patient care associate
PCS	patient classification system
PDCA	Plan Do Check Act
PDSA	Plan-Do-Study-Act
PERT	Program Evaluation and Review Technique
P-F-A	purpose-focus-approach
PHN	public health nurse

PI	performance improvement
POD	postoperative day
POS	point of service
POSDCORB	planning, organizing, supervising, directing, coordinating, reporting, and budgeting
PPO	preferred provider organization
QI	quality improvement
RN	registered nurse
RVU	relative value unit
SCHIP	State Children's Health Insurance Program
SPAN	Staff Planning and Action Network
SWOT	strengths, weaknesses, opportunities, threats
TB	tuberculosis
TEFRA	Tax Equity and Fiscal Responsibility Act
TEPP	Tobacco Education and Prevention Program
TQI	total quality improvement
UAP	unlicensed assistive personnel
UC	ubiquitous computing
URL	universal resource locator
USDHHS	United States Department of Health and Human Services
UTI	urinary tract infection
VA	Veterans Affairs
VAK	visual, auditory, kinesthetic
VR	virtual reality
WHO	World Health Organization
WOC nurse	wound, ostomy, continence nurse
WWW	World Wide Web

Appendix J: Glossary

360-degree feedback   System in which an individual is assessed by a variety of people in order to provide a broader perspective.

401K   Account that both employee and for-profit employer contribute to.

403b   Account that both employee and not-for-profit employer contribute to.

accommodating   Satisfying the needs of others, sometimes at the expense of self.

accountability   Liability for actions.

accounting   Activity that nurse managers engage in to record and report financial transactions and data.

acculturation   Process by which individuals adjust and adapt either to their host culture or a subculture by altering their own cultural behaviors.

achievement   Accomplishment of goals through effort.

activities of daily living   Activities related to toileting, bathing, grooming, dressing, feeding, mobility, and verbal and written personal communication.

activity log   Time management technique to assist in determining how time is used by periodically recording activities.

administrative law   Body of law created by administrative agencies in the form of rules, regulations, orders, and decisions to protect the rights of citizens.

administrative principles   General principles of management that are relevant to any organization.

affective domain   Learning domain centered on attitudes, or what the learner feels and believes.

affiliation   Associations and relationships with others.

agnostic   Person who is not committed to belief in the existence or nonexistence of a god or a supreme being, or perhaps believes that no one has effectively proven that a god exists.

altruism   The unselfish concern for the welfare of others.

American Nurses Association   Full-service professional organization representing the nation's entire registered nurse population.

assault   Offer to or threat of touching another in an offensive manner without that person's permission.

atheist   Does not believe in the existence of a god or a supreme being.

attending   Active listening to gain an understanding of the patient's message.

auditory   Pertaining to hearing.

authority   Power and/or right to make decisions.

autocratic leadership   Centralized decision-making style with the leader making decisions and using power to command and control others.

autonomy   An individual's right to self-determination; individual liberty.

avoiding   Retreating.

battery   Touching of another person without that person's consent.

behavioral objective   Statement of specific and measurable behavior that should result from the teaching session.

benchmark   A quantitative or qualitative standard or point of reference used in measuring or judging quality or value.

benchmarking   Management tool for seeking out the best practices in one's industry so as to improve performance.

beneficence   The duty to do good to others and to maintain a balance between benefits and harms.

bioethics   Ethics specific to health care; serves as a framework to guide behavior in ethical dilemmas.

break-even point   That point at which income and expenses are equal.

budget   A plan that provides formal quantitative expression for acquiring and distributing funds over the ensuing time period.

bureaucratic organization   Hierarchy with clear superior-subordinate communication and relations, based on positional authority, in which orders from the top are transmitted down through the organization via a clear chain of command.

capital budget   Accounts for the purchase of major new or replacement equipment.

capitation   Payment of a fixed dollar amount, per person, for the provision of health services to a patient population for a specified period of time (e.g., one month).

care delivery model   Method to organize the work of caring for patients.

case management   Strategy to improve patient care and reduce hospital costs through coordination of care.

certification   Process by which a non-governmental agency or association asserts that an individual licensed to practice a profession has met certain predetermined standards specified by that profession for practice.

certified registered nurse anesthetist   Advanced clinical nursing specialist who manages the patient's anesthesia needs before, during, and after surgery or other procedures in conjunction with other health care professionals.

change   Making something different from what it was.

change agent   One who is responsible for implementation of a change project.

civil law   That body of law that governs how individuals relate to each other in everyday matters.

clarifying   Restating, rephrasing, or questioning a message as part of a process to help make meaning clear.

clinical information system (CIS)   Collection of software programs and associated hardware that supports the entry, retrieval, update, and analysis of patient care information and associated clinical information related to patient care.

clinical ladder   A promotional model that acknowledges that staff members have varying skill sets based on their education and experience. As such, depending on skills and experience, staff members may be rewarded differently and carry differing responsibilities for patient care and the governance and professional practice of the work unit.

clinical nurse specialist   Advanced practice registered nurse, with either a master's or doctoral degree in a clinical specialty, who functions as health care provider, educator, consultant, researcher, and leader.

clinical pathway   Care management tool that outlines the expected clinical course and outcomes for a specific patient type.

cognitive domain   Learning domain centered on knowledge, or what the learner knows.

collaborating   Resolving conflict so that both parties are satisfied.

collective action   Method to deal with problems by acting as a group with a single voice.

collective bargaining   Practice of employees, in a collective group, bargaining with management in reference to wages, work practice, and other benefits.

collective bargaining agent   Individual who works with employees to formalize collective bargaining though unionization.

committee   Work group with a specific task or goal to accomplish.

common law   Body of law that develops from precedents set by judicial decisions that, over time, have the force of law, as distinguished from legislative enactments.

competing   Engaging in rivalry to meet a goal.

compromising   Finding a middle ground solution where neither party gets all they want.

computer literacy   The knowledge and understanding of computers combined with the ability to use them effectively.

computerized patient record (CPR)   Electronic record that includes all information about an individual's lifetime health status and health care; replacement for the paper medical record as the primary source of information for health care, meeting all clinical, legal, and administrative requirements.

conflict   Disagreement about something of importance to each person involved.

confronting   To work jointly with others to resolve a problem or conflict

connection power   Extent to which nurses are connected with others having power.

consensus   Situation in which all group members agree to live with and support a decision, regardless of whether they totally agree.

consideration   Activities that focus on the employee and emphasize relating and getting along with people.

constitution   A set of basic laws that specifies the powers of the various segments of the government and how these segments relate to each other.

construction budget   Developed when renovation or new structures are planned.

contingency theory   Style that acknowledges that other factors in the environment influence outcomes as much as leadership style and that leader effectiveness is contingent upon or depends upon something other than the leader's behavior.

contract law   Rules that regulate certain transactions between individuals and/or legal entities such as businesses. Also governs transactions between businesses.

cost center   Departmental subsection or unit for tracking of financial data.

culture   Behaviors, norms, belief sets, values, race, traditions, and folkways of a specific group.

dashboard   Documentation tool providing a snapshot image of pertinent information and activity reflecting a point in time.

data capture   Collection and entry of data into a computer system.

decision making   Behavior exhibited in making a selection and implementing a course of action from alternatives.

defamation   Intentionally false communication, either published or publicly spoken.

delegation   Transferring to a competent individual the authority to perform a selected nursing task in a selected situation (NSCBN, 1995).

Delphi technique   Process groups employ to arrive at a decision, though group members never meet face to face; questionnaires are distributed for opinions, then summarized and disseminated with the summaries given to group members until consensus is achieved.

democratic leadership   Style in which participation is encouraged and authority is delegated to others.

deontology   Theory stating that, in determining the ethics of a situation, a person must consider the motives of the actor, not the consequences of the act.

department clinical information system   System that meets the operational needs of a particular department, such as the laboratory, radiology, pharmacy, medical records, or billing.

diagnostic-related groups   Patient groupings established by the federal government for reimbursement purposes; these groupings are sorted by patient disease or condition.

differentiated nursing practice   Care delivery model that sorts the roles, functions, and work of registered nurses according to some identified criteria, commonly education, clinical experience, and competence.

direct care   Time spent providing hands-on care to patients.

direct cost   Cost directly related to patient care within a manager's unit.

direct expenses   Expenses that are directly associated with patient care (e.g., medical and surgical supplies and drugs).

disease management   Systematic, population-based approach to identify persons at risk, intervene with specific program of care, and measure clinical and other outcomes (Epstein and Sherwood, 1996)

economics   Study of how scarce resources are allocated among possible uses.

egoism   The tendency to be self-centered or to consider only oneself and one's own interests.

emotional health   How we are feeling in relation to some type of event.

employee-centered leadership   Style with a focus on the human needs of subordinates.

empowerment   Process by which we facilitate the participation of others in decision making and take action within an environment where there is an equitable distribution of power.

enabling objective   Objective that identifies secondary behaviors that contribute to, or enable, achievement of terminal objectives.

enterprise   An organization of any size established as a business venture.

episodic care unit   Unit that sees patients for defined episodes of care; examples include dialysis or ambulatory care units.

ethical dilemma   A conflict between two or more ethical principles for which there is no correct decision.

ethics   The doctrine that the general welfare of society is the proper goal of an individual's actions rather than egoism; the branch of philosophy that concerns the distinction between right from wrong on the basis of a body of knowledge, not just on the basis of opinions.

ethnicity   Component of cultural identity that includes several factors such as race, geographic identity, physical features, and language.

ethnocentrism   Belief that one's own culture or ethnic group is better than all other groups.

evaluation   Process of determining the success of teaching; it can measure the patient's learning and the teaching's effectiveness.

evidence-based care   Recognized by nursing, medicine, health care institutions, and health policy makers as care based on state-of-the-art science reports. It is a process approach to collecting, reviewing, interpreting, critiquing, and evaluating research and other relevant literature for direct application to patient care.

evidence-based medicine   Means to integrate individual clinical medical experience with external clinical evidence using a systematic research approach (Sackett, Rosenberg, Gray, Haynes, & Richardson, 1996).

evidence-based nursing practice Conscientious, explicit, and judicious use of theory-derived, research-based information in making decisions about care delivery to individuals or groups of individuals and in consideration of individual needs and preferences (Ingersoll, 2000, p. 152).

evidence-based practice   Conscientious, explicit, and judicious use of current best evidence in making decisions about the care of individual patients (Sackett, et al., 1996, p. 71).

expert power   Power derived from the knowledge and skills nurses possess.

false imprisonment   Occurs when people are incorrectly led to believe they cannot leave a place.

fee for service reimbursement Reimbursement based on services provided.

feedback   A new message generated by the receiver in response to the original message from the sender.

fidelity   The principle of promise keeping; the duty to keep one's promise or word.

fixed costs   Expenses that are constant and are not related to productivity or volume.

focus groups   Small groups of individuals selected because of a common characteristic (e.g., a specific patient population, patients in day surgery, new diabetics, and so on) who are invited to meet in a group and respond to questions about a topic in which they are expected to have interest or expertise.

formal leadership   When a person is in a position of authority or in a sanctioned role within an organization that connotes influence.

full-time equivalent   Measure of the work commitment of a full-time employee.

functional health status   Ability to care for oneself and meet one's human needs.

functional nursing   Care delivery model that divides the nursing work into functional units that are then assigned to one of the team members.

goal   Specific aim or target that the unit wishes to attain within the time span of 1 year.

Good Samaritan laws   Laws that have been enacted to protect the health care professional from legal liability for actions rendered in an emergency when the professional is giving service without pay.

grapevine   An informal communication channel where information moves quickly and is often inaccurate.

grievance   Situation in which a union member believes that management has failed to meet the terms of the contract or labor agreement and communicates this to management.

group process Stages that a group progresses through as it matures, consisting of the following: forming, storming, norming, performing, and adjourning.

Hawthorne effect Phenomenon of being observed or studied, which results in changes in behavior.

health State of complete physical, social, and mental well-being, and not merely the absence of disease or infirmity (World Health Organization, 1998).

health determinants Biological, psychosocial, environmental (physical and social), and health system factors or etiologies that may cause changes in the health status of individuals, families, groups, populations, and communities.

health-related quality of life Those aspects of life that are influenced either positively or negatively by one's health status and health risk factors.

health risk factors Modifiable and non-modifiable variables that increase or decrease the probability of illness or death; synonym is health determinants.

health status Level of health of an individual, family, group, population, or community; the sum of existing health risk factors, level of wellness, existing diseases, functional health status, and quality of life.

horizontal integration Occurs when a health care system contains several organizations of one type, such as hospitals.

indirect care Time spent on activities that are patient related but are not done directly to the patient.

indirect cost Cost not explicitly related to patient care within a manager's unit.

indirect expenses Expenses that are referred to such items as utilities, such as gas, electric, and phones, that are not directly related to patient care.

informal leader Individual who demonstrates leadership outside the scope of a formal leadership role or as a member of a group, rather than the head or leader of the group.

information communication Interoperability of systems and linkages for exchange of data across disparate systems.

information power Nurses who influence others with the information they provide to the group are using information power.

initiating structure Style that involves an emphasis on the work to be done, a focus on the task and production.

inpatient unit Hospital unit that is able to provide care to patients 24 hours a day, 7 days a week.

instrumental activities of daily living Activities related to food preparation and shopping; cleaning; laundry; home maintenance; verbal, written, and electronic community communications; financial management; and transportation, as well as activities to meet social and support needs, manage health care needs, access community services and resources, and meet spiritual needs.

integrated delivery system Network of health care organizations that provides a coordinated continuum of service to a defined population and is willing to be held clinically and fiscally accountable for the outcomes and the health status of the population served. Networks include hospitals, nursing homes, schools, public health departments, and social and community health organizations.

intellectual health Activities that maintain intellectual curiosity; consists of the knowledge we accumulate and the ability to think.

interdisciplinary team Group composed of members with a variety of clinical expertise.

interpersonal communication Concerned with communication between individuals.

intrapersonal communication Self-talk.

job-centered leaders Style that focuses on schedules, cost, and efficiency with less attention to developing work groups and high-performance goals.

justice The principle of fairness that is served when an individual is given that which he or she is due, owed, deserves, or can legitimately claim.

kinesthetic Pertaining to touching.

knowledge workers Those involved in serving others through their specialized knowledge.

laissez-faire leadership Passive and permissive style in which the leader defers decision making.

leader-member relations Feelings and attitudes of followers regarding acceptance, trust, and credibility of the leader.

leadership Process of influence whereby the leader influences others toward goal achievement.

learner analysis Process of identifying the learner's unique characteristics and needs.

learning domains Taxonomies, or classifications, of learning.

learning style Particular manner in which an individual responds to and processes learning.

legitimate power Power derived from the position a nurse holds in a group; it indicates the nurse's degree of authority.

lesson plan Document that provides the blueprint for the teaching session; it lists the objectives, topics, format, strategies, materials, and evaluation used in the teaching session.

living will Document voluntarily signed by patients that specifies the type of care they desire if and when they are in a terminal state and cannot sign a consent form or convey this information verbally.

maintenance or hygiene factors (Herzberg) Elements such as salary, job security, working conditions, status, quality of supervision, and relationships with others that prevent job dissatisfaction.

malpractice Professional's wrongful conduct in discharge of professional duties or failure to meet standards of care for the profession, which results in harm to another individual entrusted to the professional's care.

management Process of coordinating actions and allocating resources to achieve organizational goals.

management process Function of planning, organizing, coordinating, and controlling.

margin Profit.

MEDLARS (Medical Literature Analysis and Retrieval System) Computerized system of databases and databanks offered by the National Library of Medicine.

message Originating with the sender, consists of verbal and nonverbal stimuli that are taken in by the receiver.

methodology Structured, standardized approach for developing teaching.

mission Call to live out something that matters or is meaningful; an organization's mission reflects the purpose and direction of the health care agency or a department within it.

mission statement A formal expression of the purpose or reason for existence of the organization.

modular nursing Care delivery model that is a kind of team nursing that divides a geographical space into modules of patients with each module having a team of staff led by an RN to care for them.

money market account Similar to a bank checking account though it often requires a larger minimum amount of money to open the account and often has a higher interest rate for your money.

morality Behavior in accordance with custom or tradition; usually reflects personal or religious beliefs.

motivation Whatever influences our choices and creates direction, intensity, and persistence in our behavior.

motivation factors (Herzberg) Elements such as achievement, recognition, responsibility, advancement, and the opportunity for development that all contribute to job satisfaction.

negligence Failure to provide the care a reasonable person would ordinarily provide in a similar situation.

networking Continuous process of initiating and maintaining professional relationships through communication and information sharing.

Nonmaleficence The principle of doing no harm.

nonproductive hours Paid time not devoted to patient care; includes benefit time such as vacation, sick time, and education time.

nonverbal communication Aspects of communication that are outside what is spoken.

nurse practitioner Advanced practice nurse who has education beyond the bachelor's degree in a clinical specialty area strongly focused on primary care, though two subspecialties are hospital based (NNP and ACNP).

nursing hours per patient day Standard measure that quantifies the nursing time available to each patient by the available nursing staff.

objective Measurable step that must be taken to reach a goal.

operational budget Account for the income and expenses associated with day-to-day activity within a department or organization.

optimal outcomes Best possible objectives to be achieved given the resources at hand.

organizational change Planned alteration in an organization to generally improve efficiency.

outcome elements of quality Outcome elements of quality are the end products of quality care; outcomes review the status of patients that may result from health care. Outcome elements ask the question, "Is the patient better as a result of health care?

Pareto principle Principle, developed by Pareto, a 19th century economist, which states that 20% of effort results in 80% of results, or conversely that 80% of unfocused effort results in 20% of results.

patient acuity Measure of nursing workload that is generated for each patient.

patient care redesign Initiative in the 1990s to redesign how care was delivered.

patient-centered care Care delivery model in which care and services are brought to the patient.

patient classification system (PCS) System for distinguishing among different patients based on their acuity, functional ability, or resource needs.

patient-focused care A model of differentiated nursing practice that emphasizes quality, cost, and value.

patient-focused clinical information system System in which automation supports patient care processes; typical applications include order entry, results reporting, clinical documentation, care planning, and clinical pathways.

payer Third-party reimburser (insurance company or government).

performance improvement Structured system for creating organization-wide participation and partnership in planning and implementing continuous improvement methods to understand and meet or exceed customer needs and expectations.

personal change Alteration made voluntarily for one's own reasons, usually for self-improvement.

philosophy Statement of beliefs based on core values; rational investigations of the truths and principles of knowledge, reality, and human conduct.

philosophy of an organization A value statement of the principles and beliefs that direct the organization's behavior

physical health Encompasses nutrition and exercise coupled with a balanced amount of rest; health preventive behaviors such as avoiding smoking; and health screening behaviors that detect health problems early such as an annual Pap smear.

political voice An increase in the number of voices supporting or opposing an issue.

politics Process by which people use a variety of methods to achieve their goals.

population-based health care practice Development, provision, and evaluation of multidisciplinary health care services to population groups experiencing increased health risks or disparities, in partnership with health care consumers and the community in order to improve the health of the community and its diverse population groups.

population-based nursing practice Practice of nursing in which the focus of care is to improve the health status of vulnerable or at-risk population groups within the community by employing health promotion and disease prevention interventions across the health continuum.

position power Degree of formal authority and influence associated with the leader.

power Ability to create, get, and use resources to achieve one's goals.

power of attorney Legal document executed by an individual (principal) granting another person (agent) the right to perform certain activities in the principal's name.

practice guideline Descriptive tool or standardized specifications for care of the typical patient in the typical situation; these guidelines are developed by a formal process that incorporates the best scientific evidence of effectiveness and expert opinion. Synonyms or near synonyms include practice parameter, preferred practice pattern, algorithm, protocol, and clinical standard (JCAHO, 1999, p. 113).

preferred provider organization (PPO) Contracts with health care providers (physicians and hospitals) and payers (self-insured employers, insurance companies, government, or managed care organizations) to provide health care services to a defined population for predetermined, fixed fees.

primary health care Services that emphasize the promotion of health and the prevention of illness or disability.

primary nursing Care delivery model that clearly delineates the responsibility and accountability of the RN and places the RN as the primary provider of nursing care to patients.

problem solving Active process that starts with a problem and ends with a solution.

process Set of causes and conditions that repeatedly come together in a series of steps to transfer inputs into outcomes.

process elements of quality Identify what nursing and health care interventions must be in place to deliver quality.

Process elements are such things as managing the health care process, utilizing clinical practice guidelines and standards for nursing and medical interventions, passing medications, and so on.

productive hours   Hours worked and available for patient care.

professional change   Alteration made in position or job such as obtaining education or credentials.

professional health   Satisfaction with career choice and belief in continuous opportunity for growth.

profit   Determined by the relationship of income to expenses.

progressive discipline   System in which the manager and employee's mutual goal is to take steps to correct performance in order to bring it back to an acceptable level; it offers a stepwise process with opportunities for continued feedback and clarification of expectations.

protective factors   Patient strengths and resources that the patients can use to combat health threats that compromise core human functions.

psychomotor domain   Learning domain centered on skills, or what the learner does.

public law   General classification of law, consisting generally of constitutional, administrative, and criminal law. Public law defines a citizen's relationship with government.

quality assurance   Inspection approach to ensure that minimum standards of care exist in health care institutions, primarily hospitals.

quality improvement   Systematic process to improve outcomes based on customers' needs.

quality of life   Level of satisfaction one has with the actual conditions of one's life, including satisfaction with socioeconomic status, education, occupation, home, family life, recreation, and the ability to enjoy life, freedom, and independence.

reasonable outcomes   Objectives that can and should be achieved given less-than-optimal circumstances and limited resources.

receiver   One who takes in a message and analyzes it.

reengineering   Turning an organization upside down and inside out through fundamental rethinking and radical redesign of processes to achieve dramatic improvements in critical performance.

referent power   Power derived from how much others respect and like any individual, group, or organization.

reflective thinking   Watching or observing ourselves as we perform a task or make a decision about a certain situation.

relative value unit (RVU)   Index number assigned to various health care services based on the relative amount of resources (labor and capital) used to produce the service.

religion   Organized and public belief system of worship and practices that generally has a focus of a god or supernatural power.

resilience   The social and psychosocial capacity of individuals and groups to adapt, succeed, and persereve over time in the face of recurring threats to psychosocial and physiologic integrity.

resources   People, money, facilities, technology, and rights to properties, services, and technologies.

respect for others   Acknowledgement of the right of people to make their own decisions.

responding   Verbally and nonverbally acknowledging a sender's message.

responsibility   Reliability, dependability, and the obligation to accomplish work.

resume Brief summary of your background, training, and experience as well as your qualifications for a position.

revenue Income generated through a variety of means (e.g., billable patient services, investments, and donations to the organization).

reward/coercive power Power to reward or punish others, as well as power to instill fear in others to influence them to change their behavior; withholding rewards or achieving a goal by causing others to fear often results in resentment.

risk adjustment Process of statistically adjusting patient data to reflect significant patient variables.

Roth IRA Individual retirement account that is much less restrictive than an IRA; first introduced in 1998.

secondary health care Services that emphasize detection and early intervention in illness to prevent further illness and disability.

self-scheduling Process in which staff on a unit collectively decide and implement the monthly work schedule.

sentinel event Unexpected occurrence involving death or serious physical or psychological injury to a patient.

shared governance Situation where nurses and managers work together to define their roles and expected outcomes, holding everyone accountable for their role and expected outcomes.

shift action plan Written plan based on a shift assessment that includes a global perspective and sets the priorities for the accomplishment of outcomes that are both optimal and reasonable.

situational leadership A framework that maintains that there is no one best leadership style, but rather that effective leadership lies in matching the appropriate leadership style to the individual's or group's level of motivation and task-relevant readiness.

skill mix Percentage of RN staff to other direct care staff, LPNs, and UAP.

social health Ability to relate to and interact with others.

sources of power Combination of conscious and unconscious factors that allow an individual to influence others to do as the individual wants.

spiritual Refers to a belief in a higher power, an awareness of life and its meaning, the centering of a person with purpose in life.

spiritual distress Questioning of the purpose of life and its meaning, refusing to participate in one's usual religious practices, and seeking unusual assistance rather than the usual spiritual or religious support.

spiritual health Human capacity to find strength from within; results from a connection with a higher being or power (Chilton, 1998).

staffing pattern Plan that articulates how many and what kind of staff are needed, by shift and day, to staff a unit or department.

stakeholder Provider, employer, customer, patient, or payer who may have an interest in, and seek to influence, the decisions and actions of an organization.

stakeholders Vested interest groups.

stakeholder assessment A systematic consideration of all potential stakeholders to ensure that the needs of each of these stakeholders are incorporated in the planning phase.

storage Physical location of data in a CPR.

strategic plan The sum total or outcome of the processes by which an organization engages in environmental analysis, goal formulation and strategy development with the purpose of organizational growth and renewal.

strategic planning A process that is designed to achieve goals in dynamic, competitive environments through the allocation of resources.

structure elements of quality Identify what structures must be in place in a health care system/unit to deliver quality health care. Structure elements consist of such things as a well constructed hospital, quality patient care standards, quality staffing policies, environmental standards, and the like.

substitutes for leadership Variables that may influence or have an effect on followers to the same extent as the leader's behavior.

SWOT analysis A tool that is frequently used to conduct environmental assessments. SWOT stands for Strengths, Weaknesses, Opportunities, and Threats.

system Interdependent group of items, people, or processes with a common purpose.

task structure Involves the degree that work is defined, with specific procedures, explicit directions and goals.

team Small number of people with complementary skills who are committed to a common purpose, performance goals and approach for which they hold themselves accountable (Katzenbach & Smith, 1993).

team nursing Care delivery model that assigns staff to teams that then are responsible for a group of patients.

teleology Theory stating that the value of a situation is determined by its consequences; the outcome of an action, not the action itself, is the criterion for measuring the goodness of that action.

terminal objective Objective that identifies major behaviors that contribute to achievement of the overall session goal.

tertiary health care Services that provide restorative or rehabilitation services for patients with chronic or irreversible conditions.

Theory X View that in bureaucratic organizations, employees prefer security, direction, and minimal responsibility; coercion, threats, or punishment are necessary because people do not like the work to be done.

Theory Y View that in the context of the right conditions, people enjoy their work, they can show self-control and discipline, are able to contribute creatively and are motivated by ties to the group, the organization, and the work itself; belief that people are intrinsically motivated by their work.

Theory Z View of collective decision making and a focus on long-term employment that involves slower promotions and less direct supervision.

time management Set of related common-sense skills that helps you use your time in the most effective and productive way possible. (Mind Tools, n.d.-b)

tort A private or civil wrong or injury, including action for bad faith breach of contract, for which the court will provide a remedy in the form of an action for damages.

total patient care Care delivery model in which nurses are responsible for the total care for their patient assignment for the shift they are working.

traditional IRA Individual retirement account.

transcultural nursing Comparative study and analysis of different cultures and subcultures in the world with respect to their caring behavior, nursing care and health-illness values, beliefs, and patterns of behavior with the goal of developing a scientific and humanistic body of knowledge to provide culture-specific and culture-universal nursing care practices (Leininger, 1997).

transformational leader Leader who is committed to a vision that empowers others.

ubiquitous computing   Term coined by Mark Weiser of Xerox PARC, it describes the phase of computing in which there are many computers to one person.

union   Formal and legal group that works through a collective bargaining agent and within the context of the National Labor Relations Board to bring forth workers' requests to management.

values   Personal beliefs about the truth of ideals, standards, principles, objects, and behaviors that give meaning and direction to life.

variable costs   Costs that vary with volume and will increase or decrease depending on the number of patients.

variance   Difference between what was budgeted and the actual cost.

veracity   The obligation to tell the truth.

verbal communication   Aspect of communication that relies on spoken words to convey a message.

vertical integration   Occurs when different stages of health care are linked and delivered by one agency.

visual   Pertaining to seeing.

voting block   Group that represents the same political position or perspective.

vulnerable population groups   Subgroups of a community that are powerless, marginalized, or disenfranchised and are experiencing health disparities.

whistle-blowing   Act in which an individual discloses information regarding a violation of a law, rule or regulation or a substantial and specific danger to public health or safety.

workplace advocacy   Activities nurses undertake to address problems in their everyday workplace setting.

Code Legend

NP	Phases of the Nursing Process
As	Assessment
An	Analysis
Pl	Planning
Im	Implementation
Ev	Evaluation

CN	Client Need
Sa	Safe Effective Care Environment
Sa/1	Management of Care
Sa/2	Safety and Infection Control
He/3	Health Promotion and Maintenance
Ps/4	Psychosocial Integrity
Ph	Physiological Integrity
Ph/5	Basic Care and Comfort
Ph/6	Pharmacological and Parenteral Therapies
Ph/7	Reduction of Risk Potential
Ph/8	Physiological Adaptation

CL	Cognitive Level
K	Knowledge
Co	Comprehension
Ap	Application
An	Analysis

SA	Subject Area
1	Medical-Surgical
2	Psychiatric and Mental Health
3	Maternity and Women's Health
4	Pediatric
5	Pharmacologic
6	Gerontologic
7	Community Health
8	Legal and Ethical Issues

Practice Test 1

1. An Asian-American client is encouraged to drink fluids after undergoing an angiogram. The nurse offers the client ice cold water but the client refuses. The nurse views this behavior as

   1. manipulative and controlling.
   2. disrespectful.
   3. cultural preference.
   4. misunderstanding postprocedure routines.

2. The family of an African-American client has requested a chaplain visit while the client is in surgery. The family members speak loudly, are overflowing into the hallway, and are hugging and crying frequently. The nurse evaluates this behavior as

   1. reflecting common characteristics consistent with the African-American culture.
   2. inappropriate display of emotions.
   3. an extended support network acting inappropriately.
   4. an excuse for everyone to get together.

3. A Hispanic-American client has been diagnosed with diabetes mellitus. The client is receiving nutritional education from the diabetes nurse educator. Which statement by the client indicates an understanding of the diabetes teaching?

   1. "I will continue to eat beans, rice, and tortillas."
   2. "I enjoy deep fried burritos."
   3. "When I am busy, I purchase fast food."
   4. "I eat some kind of dessert each evening."

4. The urgent care nurse is preparing to assess a Hispanic-American child brought in by the mother. The mother states the child has been coughing. During the assessment of the child, the nurse should avoid which of the following?

    1. Taking the blood pressure

    2. Assessing lung sounds

    3. Asking the mother about immunizations

    4. Admiring the child

5. The nurse educator providing an in-service class on cultural diversity was asked to explain what cultural diversity means. Which statement by the nurse educator best describes cultural diversity?

    1. Broad information about a culture and its traditions

    2. Basic assumptions or personal convictions about a culture

    3. The process of learning norms, beliefs, and behavioral expectations of a group

    4. The differences in values, beliefs, norms, and practices between cultures

6. A Hispanic-American client mentioned to the nurse that later in the day a curandero would be visiting. The nurse understands a curandero to be which of the following?

    1. A kinship support network

    2. A folk healer.

    3. A religious figure from the church community

    4. A sacred individual specializing in the use of aromatherapy

7. A nursing student was asked to describe the meaning of cultural competency during postclinical conference. Which of the following statements by the student most appropriately describes the importance of cultural competency in planning the client's care?

    1. "A sense of understanding another culture other than one's own culture."

    2. "An extended study of a specific culture, typically within the context of the particular group."

    3. "Having knowledge, understanding, and skills regarding a diverse culture."

    4. "The differences in values, beliefs, norms, and practices among cultures."

8. The community health nurse is working with an American Indian group on nutrition education. Which of the following American Indian dietary practices should the nurse include in the plan of care?

1. The diet consists mainly of meats
2. Fruits and vegetables are staples
3. Lactose intolerance is a concern
4. Corn is not frequently consumed

9. A traditional healer of American Indians is a medicine man or woman. The nurse defines the philosophy of this practice based on which of the following?

   1. The interrelationship of human beings, the earth, and the universe.
   2. The selection of the medicine man or woman by the tribal leader.
   3. The completion of training through a certification program.
   4. The utilization of medications available through special pharmacies.

10. An Arab-American client recovering from a cholecystectomy refuses to ambulate. The nurse explains the benefits of postoperative exercise but the client continues to refuse. The nurse documents this as

    1. an expectation that the pain will be too unbearable during activity.
    2. a lack of understanding of the benefits of exercise.
    3. a cultural belief in conserving energy for recovery.
    4. a fear of physical harm with activity.

11. A nurse is caring for an American Indian client in the medical-surgical unit. The nurse asks the client to remove the metal pin attached to her gown prior to an MRI. The client refuses stating, "This is what keeps me alive; without this, my spirit is dead." Which of the following is the most appropriate response by the nurse?

    1. "Let me notify the physician of your refusal to remove the pin."
    2. " I will call the diagnostic area to reschedule the test."
    3. "The charge nurse will be in to talk to you about the test."
    4. "Is there another sacred symbol you could take to the test?"

12. The nurse is collecting a nursing history on an Arab-American client. When discussing health and illness beliefs, the nurse should consider which of the following traditional Arab-American beliefs in the plan of care?

    1. A focus on wellness and wholeness
    2. A person is healthy if at peace from within
    3. Nature, environment, and space are interrelated determinants of health and illness
    4. A belief that God or the prophet Mohammed is omnipotent and the basis for all health and illness

13. A Russian-American client has been waiting 45 minutes for a scheduled appointment at the clinic. The client is upset when the nurse begins the admission assessment. Which of the following is the most appropriate response by the nurse?

   1. "The waiting process is part of the day you can expect."
   2. "You seem frustrated; can you explain why you feel this way?"
   3. "Scheduling clinic appointments is a very complicated process."
   4. "I can't stand waiting for my clinic appointments either."

14. The research nurse at a community clinic is asked by a staff nurse to describe what an "emic" viewpoint is. Which of the following is the most appropriate response by the research nurse?

   1. "A person's way of describing an action or event, an inside view."
   2. "A fixed notion or an idea that eliminates individuality."
   3. "An interpretation of an event by someone who is not experiencing that event."
   4. "A principle that has cultural significance to a certain group."

15. An American Indian is being evaluated at the clinic with complaints of dizziness and heart palpitations. The nurse reviewing the client's laboratory values identifies several electrolyte imbalances. Which of the following American Indian remedies does the nurse assess as responsible for the electrolyte imbalances?

   1. Stargazing
   2. Divination
   3. Aromatherapy
   4. Purification

16. The nurse asks another nurse why an Arab-American client has refused all meals and fluids during the morning, afternoon, and early evening hour. The appropriate response by the nurse is that "the client

   1. is giving up hope and has started refusing nourishment."
   2. is demonstrating an ability to control the situation by refusing meals."
   3. is following fasting rituals consistent with Ramadan."
   4. is frustrated with the quality of food available."

17. A nursing instructor has asked a student nurse to describe acculturation. Which of the following is the most appropriate response by the student nurse?

   1. "The belief that one's own culture is superior to all others."
   2. "The process of acquiring norms, beliefs, and behavioral expectations of a group."

3. "The interpretation of an event by someone who is not experiencing that event."

4. "Values, beliefs, norms, and practices of a particular group."

18. A Russian-American client is attending nutritional counseling for difficulties associated with obesity. The nurse explains the importance of maintaining a healthy body weight. The client states, "I don't need to know this information. My weight has been this way for a long time and I will deal with it later." The nurse should report this as which of the following?

    1. A denial about the weight problem

    2. A tactic to control the situation and ignore the weight issue

    3. A response parallel to the Russian-American culture's time perspective

    4. A feeling of frustration with the current weight issue

19. The nurse is admitting an Arab-American client for a hernia repair. There are several people with the client and the admission room is quite small. Which of the following is the most appropriate action for the nurse to take?

    1. Insist that all but two people leave the admission room

    2. Explain that there are restrictions to the number of people allowed in the admissions area

    3. Continue with the admission process

    4. Postpone the admission until the visitors leave

20. The hospice nurse caring for a terminally ill Arab-American client is asked by family members to reposition the bed so the client's body is facing a certain direction. Which of the following should the nurse consider before responding to this request? The client and family

    1. want a change in the scenery and environment.

    2. prefer to face Mecca to pray.

    3. are hoping for a different room.

    4. are expecting more visitors and moving the bed would allow more room.

21. The pediatric nurse is preparing immunizations for a Russian-American toddler. The toddler's mother appears anxious and is asking questions regarding the needles, syringes, and packaging. Which of the following is the most appropriate response by the nurse?

    1. "You don't need to worry, I've done this hundreds of times."

    2. "I'm afraid your anxiety could be upsetting your child."

    3. "This will be over in a matter of seconds."

    4. "You seem apprehensive about this; I will explain our procedure for immunizations."

22. The nurse is asked to describe religious and spiritual characteristics of the Russian-American culture from a historical perspective to a group of nurses. Which of the following explanations should the nurse include to the group?

    1. Prayer visits from rabbi, priests, or ministers may be requested from the client

    2. Prohibition of religion in the former Soviet Union resulted in many immigrants not practicing a faith

    3. During lent, animal and dairy products are forbidden

    4. There are some required fasting days associated with the Eastern Orthodox Church

23. The nurse is educating a Hispanic-American client about the management of hypertension. Which of the following client behaviors indicates to the nurse that the client understands the information? The client is

    1. polite and taking notes.

    2. sitting close and has direct eye contact.

    3. quiet and looking out the window.

    4. touching the blood pressure cuff.

24. The nurse will spend a year studying the lifeways of a tribe in Namibia, Africa, and live in a village with members of the community to learn about their health care needs. The nurse explains that living among the people of Namibia provides which of the following?

    1. Cohabitation

    2. Socialization

    3. Ethnocentrism

    4. Acculturation

25. The community health nurse working with American Indian families at an immunization clinic is concerned because many clients have not followed their schedule of appointments. The nurse evaluates the clients' failure to keep scheduled appointments as

    1. having a lack of understanding about the importance of immunizations.

    2. possessing a casual and flexible sense of time.

    3. lacking a respect for medical interventions.

    4. a fear of pain associated with the immunizations.

ANSWERS AND RATIONALES

1. 3. The dietary practice of many Asian-American clients involves the *yin* and *yang* beliefs. The *yin* foods are cold and *yang* foods are hot and influence balance in the body. This client could be sensing an imbalance and may prefer hot liquids at this time. The *yin* and *yang* represent a balance between positive and negative energy forces.
   NP = An
   CN = Sa/1
   CL = An
   SA = 8

2. 1. The African-American communication style is often very expressive and loud. Nonverbal communication, such as hugging and touching, are signs of affection in this culture. Extended family and close friends are considered part of the kin support network.
   NP = Ev
   CN = Sa/1
   CL = An
   SA = 8

3. 1. Typical Hispanic-American diet includes rice, beans, corn, and tortillas. These foods provide needed carbohydrates with limited amounts of fat or sugar. A Hispanic-American client who intends to continue to eat rice, beans, corn, and tortillas demonstrates an understanding of the concepts involved in controlling diabetes through nutritional management.
   NP = Ev
   CN = Sa/1
   CL = Ap
   SA = 8

4. 4. In the Hispanic-American culture, the concept of "mal ojo," or evil eye, is a belief that illness may be caused by a person with a strong eye (direct eye contact) who admires while touching the child. The Hispanic-American client is comfortable with touch.
   NP = As
   CN = Sa/1
   CL = Ap
   SA = 8

5. 4. Broad information about a culture is generalization. Basic assumptions or personal convictions that an individual believes are true are beliefs. The process of learning norms, beliefs, and behavioral expectations of a group are acculturation. Cultural diversity considers the differences between the values, beliefs, norms, and practices of a variety of cultures.

NP = Ev
CN = Sa/1
CL = Ap
SA = 8

6. 2. In times of illness, Hispanic-American clients may utilize both biomedical and folk health systems. A curandero is a folk healer in the Hispanic culture.
NP = An
CN = Sa/1
CL = Ap
SA = 8

7. 3. Cultural competency is defined as having knowledge, understanding, and skills regarding a diverse culture.
NP = Ev
CN = Sa/1
CL = An
SA = 8

8. 3. Traditional American Indian diets in the past consisted of fruits, berries, roots, fish, and game. The traditional diet has been transformed as a result of scarcity of food in federally defined Indian geographic regions. Modern, processed foods high in fat and sugar are more common. Lactose intolerance is common and many people do not drink milk.
NP = Pl
CN = Ph/5
CL = Ap
SA = 8

9. 1. American Indians believe that health is a reflection of harmony with family, environment, and universe. The medicine man may be consulted and is an important part of treatment. Certification, selection by the tribal leader, and the use of special pharmacies are not part of the traditional philosophy.
NP = Im
CN = Sa/1
CL = Ap
SA = 8

10. 3. There is a strong belief in the Arab-American culture regarding rest and conserving energy for a proper recovery. This is in direct conflict with the Western practice of exercising (ambulating) to improve recovery and avoid complications. Understanding this cultural preference is important for the nurse in providing care.
NP = Im
CN = Sa/1

CL = An
SA = 8

11. 4. Symbolic or sacred items may be used for healing and blessings in the American Indian culture. Explaining the restrictions involved with certain diagnostic equipment may help the client understand the reasoning behind the request for removal. Offering to substitute the pin for another one of the symbols is a good compromise.
NP = An
CN = Sa/1
CL = An
SA = 8

12. 4. When assessing Arab-American clients, it is important to understand their strong religious foundation, as this guides their health and illness belief system. Their health and illness beliefs center on the belief that God or the prophet Mohammed is omnipotent and the basis for all health and illness. If one loses faith in God, then illness may befall that person. A person in harmony with God is healthy.
NP = Pl
CN = Sa/1
CL = An
SA = 8

13. 2. Asking for clarification or understanding in certain situations can be helpful to both the client and the nurse. In the Russian culture, punctuality is important and lateness is considered rude.
NP = An
CN = Sa/1
CL = An
SA = 8

14. 1. A person's way of describing an action or event from an inside view is an emic viewpoint. A stereotype is a fixed notion or concept of a group or person that eliminates all individuality. The interpretation of an event by someone who is not experiencing that event or from an outside view is an etic viewpoint. A value includes principles that have meaning and worth to a certain group of people.
NP = An
CN = Sa/1
CL = An
SA = 8

15. 4. The traditional American Indian remedy of purification may include immersion in water, sweat lodges, special rituals, and herbs. These practices may cause electrolyte disturbances.
NP = As
CN = Sa/1

CL = Ap
SA = 8

16. 3. Many Arab-American clients participate in fasting during the month of Ramadan. No eating, drinking, or smoking is permitted from sunrise to sunset. Meals are traditionally served at night during this month.
NP = An
CN = Sa/1
CL = An
SA = 8

17. 2. A belief that one's own culture is superior to all others is the definition of ethnocentrism. Interpreting an event by someone who is not experiencing the event, an outside view, is an etic viewpoint. Values, beliefs, norms, and practices of a particular group define that group's culture. The process of acquiring the norms, beliefs, and behavioral expectations of a particular group is acculturation.
NP = An
CN = Sa/1
CL = An
SA = 8

18. 3. The Russian-American culture typically is future oriented. People of this culture look to the future, rather than the past or present time frame. This may explain the reason the client does not want to deal with the weight issue at this time.
NP = An
CN = Sa/1
CL = An
SA = 8

19. 3. People immersed in the Arab-American culture show respect and support through their presence. This may include extended family and friends.
NP = Im
CN = Sa/1
CL = Ap
SA = 8

20. 2. Arab-American clients may be Muslim and practice religious duties consistent within this belief system. Praying five times per day while facing Mecca is one of the religious pillars of their faith.
NP = An
CN = Sa/1
CL = Ap
SA = 8

21. 4. Historically, the economy in Russia has led to severe shortages of equipment and supplies. Often supplies are reused without proper sterilization. Russian-Americans typically have great respect for Western medicine, but thorough explanations are expected.
NP = An
CN = Sa/1
CL = An
SA = 8

22. 2. Historically, religious beliefs in the Soviet Union were forbidden. The result has been that many immigrants are not participating in a certain faith.
NP = Pl
CN = Sa/1
CL = An
SA = 8

23. 1. Nonverbal communication in the Hispanic-American culture involves gestures. Eye contact is avoided with authority figures. Silence could indicate a lack of agreement.
NP = An
CN = Sa/1
CL = An
SA = 8

24. 4. Acculturation is the process of learning norms, beliefs, and behavioral expectations of a group. Living in a village or community within the group one is studying is an excellent way to gain a true understanding of the culture.
NP = Im
CN = Sa/1
CL = An
SA = 8

25. 2. Time orientation from the American Indian perspective is viewed as being on a continuum, with no beginning and no end. "Indian time" is considered flexible and casual. Many homes have no clocks.
NP = Ev
CN = Sa/1
CL = An
SA = 8

LEADERSHIP AND MANAGEMENT-COMPREHENSIVE EXAM

1. The inclement weather policy has been activated in the local hospital. The charge nurse conducts a discussion of the situation with the staff available. Which of the nursing care delivery systems is most appropriate in this situation?

   1. Team nursing

   2. Primary nursing

   3. Case management

   4. Functional nursing

ANSWERS AND RATIONALES

1. **4.** Functional nursing is efficient and requires fewer staff than other systems. It divides nursing into functional units that are assigned to one of the team members. Each team member has specific tasks or duties. Primary nursing is a model of nursing that delineates the responsibility and accountability of the client's care to the RN. In the case management model of nursing, a nurse is assigned to a specific high-risk population. Both primary nursing and case management require a large number of registered nurses. Team nursing is a model of nursing in which staff members are assigned to be responsible for the care delivered to a client. It is unlikely that staff members are available for the efficient use of skills in this model.

   NP = An

   CN = Sa/1

   CL = An

   SA = 8

Practice Test 2

1. A young couple is reviewing health care services in the community. Both are healthy and interested in staying that way. They ask the nurse which health care services would be appropriate for them. The appropriate response by the nurse is

   1. "primary care."

   2. "secondary care."

   3. "tertiary care."

   4. "rehabilitative care."

2. The nurse should instruct the parents of a son who has diabetes mellitus to bring him to which of the following local health care systems that provides health care, school activities, and camp services for clients with diabetes only?

   1. Diagnostic-related groups health care

   2. Community, school, and home health care

   3. Population-based health care

   4. Case management health care

3. The nurse working on a unit recognizes the need for total, holistic care and identifies organized, efficient, and quality delivery of care as its goal. Which of the following is most descriptive of this goal?

   1. Management of client care

   2. Management of client outcomes

   3. Quality management services

   4. Case management services

4. Which of the following is a priority for the nurse to consider when planning care for a group of clients utilizing evidenced-based practice issues?

   1. Standardized care maps are used on all of the nurse's clients.

   2. Client care is planned based on the nurse's clinical expertise and the latest research findings.

   3. Standards of care are established at the hospital level and there is little flexibility in changing them at the unit level.

   4. Client needs are assessed and individualized plans of care are developed for each client.

5. A registered nurse utilizes which of the following legal documents when delegating a client care assignment to a licensed practical nurse (LPN) on a unit where the LPN was unfamiliar with common practice?

   1. Sunset laws in the state of practice

   2. National labor relations act

   3. State board of health professionals law

   4. Nurse practice act

6. A nurse observes another nurse who failed to wipe up water that the client spilled on the floor. The nurse who observed this as a careless omission in the delivery of care should consider which of the following as the priority before reporting this?

   1. Tort law

   2. Negligence

   3. Benchmark care

   4. Nurse practice act

7. The nurse implements what laws when notifying the state of a possible chemical addiction by a peer?_____

8. A nursing student realizes that a peer student is making up vital signs and documenting false data. Which of the following should the nurse consider when reporting this behavior to the nurse faculty or nurse manager?

   1. Sense of justice

   2. Reporting laws

   3. Nurse practice act

   4. Ethical practice and principles

9. The medical team has noticed that many of the nurses on a particular unit work together collaboratively to improve client outcomes. Leadership qualities are demonstrated by nurses at all levels. Which of the following best describes the medical team's understanding of leadership?

    1. This leadership by the nurses is directly related to the leadership ability of the nurse manager

    2. These nurses must be experienced, because leadership qualities are developed over a period of time

    3. Leadership qualities can be exhibited by anyone, not just those with administrative roles

    4. The medical staff believes that client outcomes are better on this unit because of the assertiveness of the nurses

10. The nurses who work on a 30-bed surgical unit have noticed that their unit implements new and innovative client care activities long before other units in the hospital. Which of the following leadership characteristics exhibited by the nurse manager best describes this process?

    1. Knowledge and skill

    2. Interpersonal abilities

    3. Communication techniques

    4. Vision and passion

11. The nurse manager demonstrates which of the following leadership styles by asking staff members to develop a staffing plan for November through January?

    1. Participative

    2. Democratic

    3. Autocratic

    4. Laissez-faire

12. The nurse should include which of the following concepts in a management process that is implemented effectively?
Select all that apply:

    [ ] **1.** Caregiving

    [ ] **2.** Lobbying

    [ ] **3.** Planning

    [ ] **4.** Organizing

    [ ] **5.** Discharging

    [ ] **6.** Coordinating

13. Which of the following are essential for a nurse manager who is new to the managerial role to include in this position?
Select all that apply:

    [ ] **1.** Information processing

    [ ] **2.** Performance reporting

[ ] **3.** Interpersonal skills

[ ] **4.** Educational planning

[ ] **5.** Economic development

[ ] **6.** Decision making

14. The nurse considers which of the following when employing the change theory to implement a new client care procedure?

   1. With correct information, all employees usually embrace change with enthusiasm.

   2. The change process takes time and nurturing, because all humans do not move at the same pace toward the change goals.

   3. Change is inevitable in the health care delivery system, so all employees are used to its occurrence and will not experience stress.

   4. Quality client care rarely needs adjusting once it has reached a high level of efficiency and optimal outcomes.

15. A group of nurses on a unit implementing a pilot project related to standards of care for wounds have experienced staff members who can be described as having which of the following behavioral responses to change?
   Select all that apply:

   [ ] **1.** Anticipators

   [ ] **2.** Innovators

   [ ] **3.** Adaptors

   [ ] **4.** Rejectors

   [ ] **5.** Criticizers

   [ ] **6.** Doubters

16. The nurse evaluates what type of nursing practice as a model of nursing care delivery in which roles, functions, and tasks of the professional nurse are designated by a set of criteria?

   1. Criterion-referenced

   2. Differentiated

   3. Evidenced-based

   4. Transactional

17. The charge nurse incorporates which of the following sources when making effective assignments for the next shift?

   1. Seniority preferences

   2. Recent performance evaluation

   3. Personality traits

   4. Client classification data

18. Since the charge nurse is admitting a new client to the unit, the charge nurse instructed another registered nurse to assist a resident with a spinal tap. Which of the following statements best describes this action by the charge nurse?

    1. Delegation of tasks that are within another nurse's scope of practice is a legitimate role function for a charge nurse

    2. Staffing patterns should be reexamined when the charge nurse cannot assist a resident physician

    3. The charge nurse should always negotiate add-on assignments, regardless of the other circumstances on the unit

    4. Physicians expect to work directly with nurses in a leadership position

19. The nurse supervisor should inform a nurse interviewing for a nurse manager position that accountability for client care is

    1. 40 hours per week.

    2. 56 hours per week.

    3. 120 hours per week.

    4. 168 hours per week.

20. A nursing unit has been experiencing many types of interpersonal conflicts among the nurses. The nurse manager implements which of the following concepts of conflict resolution to solve these issues?
    Select all that apply:

    [ ] **1.** Authorizing

    [ ] **2.** Avoiding

    [ ] **3.** Compromising

    [ ] **4.** Confronting

    [ ] **5.** Negotiating

    [ ] **6.** Transferring blame

21. Which of the following is a priority for the nurse manager to incorporate into the components of functional teamwork in order to establish effective teams on each shift?

    1. Optimal team performance is directly related to the number of registered nurses on the team.

    2. Every team needs someone to serve in the role of coordinator, mobilizer, questioner, antagonist, and recorder.

    3. Effective teams function through the creativity, vision, and commitment of the team leader.

    4. Teams work best when team members have worked together at least six months.

22. The nurse planning discharge teaching for a teenager and family members should include which of the following strategies of therapeutic communication?

    1. Discharge teaching should be shared with the teenager and parents and include multiple feedback loops.

    2. Teenagers are not concerned with self-care, so guidelines for care should be given to the parents.

    3. Because the attention span of teenagers is short, communication of discharge plans should be shared on the day of discharge in several short sessions.

    4. Communication techniques should be changed for the teenage group and the family members.

23. The nurse includes which of the following communication skills to enhance therapeutic nurse-client relationships?
    Select all that apply:

    [ ] 1. Attending

    [ ] 2. Clarifying

    [ ] 3. Measuring

    [ ] 4. Reacting

    [ ] 5. Responding

    [ ] 6. Transforming

24. After assessing a new nurse's stress over the complexity of the workload, the nurse manager assists the new nurse to improve organizational skills and

    1. collaboration skills.

    2. procedural skills.

    3. psychomotor skills.

    4. time-management skills.

ANSWERS AND RATIONALES

1. **1.** The focus of primary care centers is to promote health and prevent illness. Annual checkups and health promoting activities are a part of the overall goal of the services. Secondary care focuses on early detection and intervention to prevent further illness and disability. Tertiary health care provides services that are restorative or rehabilitative for clients who have conditions that are chronic or irreversible.
    NP = An
    CN = Sa/1

CL = Ap
SA = 8

2. 3. By definition, population-based health care focuses on the needs of a specific population and not just on individual clients. Diagnostic-related groups health care is not a health care system. Community, school, and home health care and case management health care are also not health care systems.
NP = Im
CN = Sa/1
CL = Ap
SA = 8

3. 1. Total management of client care includes the total organized collection of activities designed to meet the needs of the client. Management of client outcomes, quality management services, and case management services are all a part of the activities that make up the total management of client care.
NP = Ev
CN = Sa/1
CL = An
SA = 8

4. 2. Evidenced-based practice is the delivery of client care based on knowledge of the clinician, standards of care, and recent research findings.
NP = Pl
CN = Sa/1
CL = An
SA = 8

5. 4. The nurse practice act in each state provides direction and guidelines for the scope of practice of all licensed personnel in the state. Sunset laws in the state of practice, national labor relations act, and state board of health professionals law do not provide regulations for health care practice.
NP = Im
CN = Sa/1
CL = Ap
SA = 8

6. 2. The most common violations of standards of care are simple omissions in reasonable, customary client care, called negligence. Tort law is a private or civil wrong or injury including action for bad faith breach of contract.
NP = An
CN = Sa/1
CL = Ap
SA = 8

7. **Reporting laws.** Reporting laws in a state provide for reporting of abusive and addictive actions on the part of professional health care providers.
NP = Im
CN = Sa/1
CL = Ap
SA = 8

8. 4. Ethical practice and principles should be considered when reporting a nursing student who is falsely reporting vital signs, because the nursing student is not a licensed care provider. Ethical practice and principles is based on a strong commitment to right and wrong relative to clinical decision making. A sense of justice would cause the reporting of this activity of the peer to be grounded in vindictiveness rather than in professional ethics. Reporting laws are provided for reporting abusive and substance impairment of professionals. The nurse practice act provides for rules and regulatory guidelines for professional practice.
NP = An
CN = Sa/1
CL = Ap
SA = 8

9. 3. Leadership qualities can be exhibited by those who do not have positions of authority. Leadership skill can develop over time, but nurses who are experienced and inexperienced both may demonstrate leadership characteristics.
NP = An
CN = Sa/1
CL = An
SA = 8

10. 4. The nurse manager most likely is exhibiting vision and passion when the nursing unit is performing new and innovative activities long before other nursing units. While knowledge and skill, interpersonal abilities, and communication techniques may be characteristics of this nurse manager, they do not address the nurse manager's leadership approach.
NP = Ev
CN = Sa/1
CL = Ap
SA = 8

11. 1. With participative leadership style, staff members collaborate with each other to achieve common goals, such as developing a staffing plan. With democratic leadership, the nurse delegates authority to others. With laissez-faire leadership, passiveness and permissiveness exist, and the leader defers decision making. With autocratic leadership, centralized

decision making is implemented by the leader who makes decisions and uses power to command and control others.

NP = Ev

CN = Sa/1

CL = Ap

SA = 8

12. **3,4,6.** Planning, organizing, and coordinating are all concepts used in the management process. Caregiving and discharging are characteristics used in the caregiver role.

NP = Im

CN = Sa/1

CL = Ap

SA = 8

13. **1,3,6.** Information processing, interpersonal skills, and decision making are all characteristics necessary in the role of the nurse manager. Performance reporting, educational planning, and economic development are characteristics that may occur with other initiatives. These skills may only be necessary for certain projects and not essential for everyday management.

NP = Im

CN = Sa/1

CL = Ap

SA = 8

14. **2.** The fact that change takes time and nurturing, because all humans do not move at the same pace toward the change goals, should be considered when utilizing the change theory to implement a new client care procedure.

NP = An

CN = Sa/1

CL = An

SA = 8

15. **2,3,4.** According to change theory, the usual human response to change is captured by those who see it as an opportunity for new innovations (innovators); those who do not particularly want to change but do it anyway (adaptors); and those who cannot accept the change and reject it (rejectors). Anticipators, criticizers, and doubters are responders who hinder the change process.

NP = Ev

CN = Sa/1

CL = Ap

SA = 8

16. 2. Differentiated nursing practice is a model of care delivery in which the nurse is assigned activities based on an established set of criteria, such as educational background, expertise, competency, and certification. Criterion-referenced nursing is a model used for performance evaluation. Evidenced-based nursing practice is a type of nurse framework for practice based on the holistic model and includes clinical expertise as well as research findings. Transactional is a leadership style.
NP = Ev
CN = Sa/1
CL = Ap
SA = 8

17. 4. Effective assignments are made based on the nurse's clinical knowledge and expertise in client care and data relative to the acuity of illness and client needs information. Seniority preferences and personality traits should never be the driving force behind assignments; however, some specific assignments may be made based on years of experience and personality issues between nurse and client. Client classification data should not be a priority with regard to client assignments, except in situations where professional development is occurring as a result of performance outcomes.
NP = Im
CN = Sa/1
CL = Ap
SA = 8

18. 1. Delegation of tasks is within the charge nurse's scope of practice. It is appropriate for the charge nurse to change assignments based on unit and client needs at a particular moment. Reexamining staffing patterns, negotiating add-on assignments, and having physicians expect to work directly with nurses in a leadership position are unreasonable actions in the context of the common goal of client care delivery. The charge nurse should be sensitive to any of these responses that may indicate a lack of team and collaborative approaches.
NP = An
CN = Sa/1
CL = An
SA = 8

19. 4. The nurse manager assumes responsibility for client care delivery 24 hours per day, seven days per week.
NP = Im
CN = Sa/1
CL = Ap
SA = 8

20. 2,3,4,5. Avoiding, compromising, confronting, and negotiating are all strategies used at some point in a conflict to try to achieve resolution. Using an authoritative approach and transferring blame from one to another will cause greater conflict.
NP = Im
CN = Sa/1
CL = Ap
SA = 8

21. 2. The roles of team members are coordinator, mobilizer, questioner, antagonist, and recorder. Effective teams have been established and function toward optimal goal achievement without registered nurses present. Team members should also demonstrate creativity, vision, and commitment to be characteristics of effective teams. It seems reasonable that the longer team members work together, the better the results; however, this is not necessarily true.
NP = Pl
CN = Sa/1
CL = An
SA = 8

22. 1. Discharge teaching should always include the adolescent and supportive others. Multiple feedback loops will provide an opportunity to clarify information that may be misunderstood and to observe return demonstrations if appropriate.
NP = Pl
CN = Sa/1
CL = An
SA = 8

23. 1,2,5. Attending, clarifying, and responding are communication techniques that serve to increase understanding of interactions. Measuring, reacting, and transforming are not related to communication skills. Reacting is a behavioral response, perhaps to a communication.
NP = Im
CN = Sa/1
CL = Ap
SA = 8

24. 4. While knowledge of collaboration, procedural, and psychomotor skills could serve to decrease the nurse's stress level, only priority setting, organization, and effective time-management skills will ultimately decrease the issues of complexity of client care issues.
NP = Im
CN = Sa/1
CL = Ap
SA = 8

ETHICAL ISSUES-COMPREHENSIVE EXAM

1. The nurse becomes angry with the nursing supervisor, quits work, and leaves the hospital during the shift. Which of the following ethical rules has the nurse violated?
   1. Fidelity
   2. Veracity
   3. Confidentiality
   4. Justice

2. The nurse correctly identifies a situation as being an ethical dilemma. Which of the following best describes why the nurse may find using an ethical decision-making tool to be useful?
   1. Because the tool will provide the right answer
   2. Using a tool will make the nurse's decision more defensible in court
   3. To systematically evaluate ethical theories and principles
   4. It is faster than going to the ethics committee

ANSWERS AND RATIONALES

1. **1.** Fidelity involves loyalty to clients and is breached if the nurse abandons them. Justice is an ethical principle that relates to equitable division of resources. Veracity is truth telling and confidentiality deals with maintaining information in confidence. None of these principles and rules is violated as much as the rule of fidelity in a case of client abandonment.
   NP = Ev
   CN = Sa/1
   CL = Ap
   SA = 8

2. **3.** There are several ethical decision-making tools a nurse may use; they all serve to help the nurse systematically evaluate the theories and principles in conflict. Ethical decision-making tools do not provide the "right" answer, as there is often no such thing in an ethical dilemma. While using a decision-making tool immediately is more expedient than waiting for the ethics committee to meet, this is not the reason to use the tool. The nurse may still consult the ethics committee regardless of whether a tool is used. Use of such a tool may help the nurse to describe how the action taken was arrived at; however, whether this would help defend a nurse's action in court is questionable.
   NP = Ev
   CN = Sa/1
   CL = An
   SA = 8

Practice Test 3

1. A nursing student conducting research for a course asks the nurse for a list of client names, addresses, and phone numbers so the student can contact them to offer them a chance to participate in the study. Which of the following is the best action by the nurse?

    1. Provide the list to the student nurse as requested

    2. Inform the student nurse that this would breach client confidentiality

    3. Tell the student nurse that nurses do not have time for that and the student will have to obtain this from the chart

    4. Give the student nurse only the names and phone numbers so the student can call and get the addresses if the client chooses to release that information

2. A client in a double room is playing the radio very loudly. When confronted by the nurse to turn it down because it is disturbing the client's roommate, the client yells, "It is my right to play my radio as loudly as I wish!" Which of the following is the best initial response by the nurse based on an understanding of the principle of autonomy?

    1. Move the roommate to another room so that the client's autonomy can be upheld

    2. Agree with the client that autonomy to play the radio must be upheld

    3. Explain to the client that one client's rights are not more important than another's

    4. Allow the client to play the radio loudly until the chair of the ethics committee can be contacted for consultation

3. A client is trying to decide whether to undergo a mastectomy or lumpectomy. She tells the nurse that she feels she has sufficient information and wants a lumpectomy, but that her husband and his mother are insisting that she have a mastectomy. Which of the following would be the best initial response by the nurse, based on an understanding of the principle of autonomy?

   1. Inform the client that it's her choice, but that women often cope better if they choose the surgery that their family supports

   2. Assess the beliefs of the husband and mother-in-law and help the client communicate her wishes to them

   3. Inform the client that she has the right to choose whatever surgery she wants regardless of her family's insistence

   4. Recommend that the client seek advocacy support from a local woman's group in order to confront her husband and mother-in-law

ANSWERS AND RATIONALES

1. **2.** Divulging the names and any other information about clients that the client has a right to assume is being held confidential, even if it is to a student or other health professional, is breaching confidentiality. Especially where research is concerned, information about clients should not be released to someone not directly involved in the client's care without the permission of the client. Therefore, it is not acceptable for the nurse to release this information, to permit the student to review the charts, or to call clients after being given their names.
   NP = Pl
   CN = Sa/1
   CL = Ap
   SA = 8

2. **3.** According to the principle of autonomy, a client's autonomy should be respected unless, in so doing, it interferes with the rights of another. Here the loud volume of the radio is conflicting with the rights of the roommate to rest comfortably. Moving the roommate may also interfere with that person's rights to be comfortable in the room to which the client is accustomed. A better solution may be to move the client causing the disturbance. While contacting the ethics committee is always an option, it is not the best initial response to this situation.
   NP = An
   CN = Sa/1
   CL = An
   SA = 8

3. 2. It is a duty of nurses to safeguard the autonomy of clients, which includes helping to control constraints on their ability to exercise their freedom of choice effectively. Telling the client to change her decision to agree with her family is adding to the constraints. Informing the client of her rights is helpful, but does nothing to understand why her spouse and mother-in-law feel the way they do, nor does it remove the constraint being placed on her. Confronting her family with an advocate may set up an adversarial situation prematurely, which is not helpful when the woman is vulnerable facing cancer and surgery, and will need her family's support. Therefore, the best response is for the nurse to assess the beliefs of the family and help the client and her family communicate in order to remove the constraint on her autonomy.

NP = An
CN = Sa/1
CL = An
SA = 8

LEGAL ISSUES FOR OLDER ADULTS-COMPREHENSIVE EXAM

1. The nurse observes an unlicensed nurse assistant (NA) regulating the intravenous infusion of an older adult receiving 5% dextrose in water. A licensed practical nurse (LPN) on the nurse's team is responsible for the client and assigned the client to the NA. Which of the following is the priority nursing intervention by the registered nurse?

1. Instruct the LPN that this action is not within the realm of responsibility of an NA

2. Immediately inform the charge nurse and complete an occurrence report

3. Confront the LPN and the NA

4. Meet with the LPN and NA to discuss the responsibility parameters of each

2. An older adult who is a resident in a long-term care facility tells the nurse, "I don't want to live like this anymore. I'm going to save my pills and take them all at once." The nurse fails to act on this information to protect the client from self-directed violence and is guilty of

1. malpractice.

2. negligence.

3. beneficence.

4. nonmaleficence.

3. The nurse observes another nurse starting an intravenous (IV) infusion on an older adult without wearing gloves. When questioned about this breach in universal precautions, the nurse replies, "Oh, I was careful. Older people don't have anything contagious anyway." Starting an IV without gloves may harm the nurse and the client. The observing nurse should report this behavior as

1. negligence.

2. failure to follow the standard of care.

3. malpractice.

4. coercion.

4. The nurse has a full workload and must reassign some of the assigned clients to unlicensed assistive personnel (UAP). The most appropriate client to assign to UAP is

1. A 76-year-old client with suspected pancreatitis and a blood sugar of 312

2. An 83-year-old client who had a cerebrovascular accident seven days ago

3. A 68-year-old client who is in severe pain with esophageal cancer

4. A 92-year-old client who is dying

5. The nurse is teaching a class on the legal issues of older adults. Which of the following should the nurse include that would not violate the client's rights and that illustrates acceptable practice?

1. Trying to forcibly restrain a client who is competent but would suffer great harm by leaving the health care facility

2. Allowing a physical therapist who is not assigned to the client to read the client's chart

3. Giving a client emergency first aid without consent

4. Keeping a nursing home resident's letters to family members in the medical chart instead of mailing them

6. A nurse serving as a legal medical expert states, "The degree of judgment and skill in nursing care which would be given by a reasonable and prudent professional nurse under similar circumstances is _____."

7. The medical order for an older adult is written, "Benadryl 25 mg p.o. for itching p.r.n." The client is restless and agitated so the nurse administers the diphenhydramine (Benadryl), which is known to have a subduing or sedating effect. Which of the following has the nurse performed?

1. Malpractice, because the medication was given for a different reason from what it was ordered for

2. An appropriate action, since the drug has a sedating effect

3. Negligence, because the nurse did not call the prescriber

4. Dereliction of duty, because the nurse did not meet the client's needs

8. Morphine 10 mg IV push every 6 hrs p.r.n. is prescribed for an older adult who is experiencing moderate pain. The client has requested the pain medication. The nurse has prepared the medication and is about to inject it into a peripheral IV line. The daughter of the client asks the nurse not to give the morphine and states, "I don't want my mom to sleep so much. Please just give her water IV. She'll think it's her morphine and be OK." The nurse should

   1. give the IV solution as asked by the client's daughter.

   2. give neither the IV solution or the morphine.

   3. explain to the daughter the nursing assessment of the client's pain and give the morphine.

   4. tell the daughter to call the physician and discuss it.

9. An 83-year-old nursing home resident fatally injures another resident at 0300. The nurse and unlicensed assistive personnel on duty at the time were outside smoking cigarettes at the time of the incident. All residents were checked before the staff went outside and were just outside the door with the door propped open. The nurse in charge is

   1. blameless because all precautions were taken.

   2. following the standard of care because the residents were checked.

   3. negligent and liable.

   4. following policy.

10. A client is admitted to room 13, but states an unwillingness to remain in the room because the number will bring bad luck. Another room is available. The nurse should

    1. leave the client in room number 13 and tell the client to adjust.

    2. serve as an advocate for the client and move the client to another room.

    3. monitor the client but avoid moving the client.

    4. not move the client because the client may expect to continue to have all demands met.

11. A 77-year-old client tells the nurse, "I can't take sulfa drugs. I'm allergic to them." The nurse administers Septra as ordered. The client develops a rash and then respiratory distress. Even though the physician ordered the

medication and the pharmacist filled the prescription, the nurse was told of an allergy to Septra and administered it anyway. The nurse is subject to discipline for

1. malpractice.
2. assault.
3. negligence.
4. battery.

12. A nurse observes a staff member transferring an older adult male client who is confused and suspected of having Alzheimer's disease to nuclear medicine for a CT scan. The client attempts to grab the transferring staff member and another staff member says, "Watch it! He's a dirty old man." The most appropriate nursing intervention is to

1. ask the staff members to talk more quietly when in areas where the public can hear.
2. inform the transferring staff member that this is defamation of the client's character.
3. encourage the staff member to assist the transferring staff member with the client.
4. hold a staff meeting on appropriate behavior around clients.

13. A nursing home resident has a small packet in a pocket of his tee shirt kept in place by a rubber band. When the nurse asks what is in the packet, the client identifies the substance as "ginger to ward off the evil eye." The nurse smells the substance and identifies it as ginger. The nurse should

1. inform the client that there is no such thing as the "evil eye."
2. instruct the client that ginger has no medicinal use.
3. take the ginger away from the client and dispose of it.
4. leave the ginger and chart the interaction with the client.

14. Which of the following is the priority nursing intervention for a 94-year-old client who lives in a long-term care facility and has suddenly become confused?

1. Ask the licensed practical nurse (LPN) to assess the client
2. Ask the unlicensed assistive person (UAP) to stay with the client
3. Ask a registered nurse to assess the client
4. Call the physician

15. A nurse does not reposition an older adult client every two hours as specified on the nursing care plan and the physician's order. The nurse's lack of action is a violation of

1. Medicare laws for the care of the older adult.
2. Medicaid laws for the care of the older adult.
3. standards of practice.
4. standardized care plans.

16. Which of the following criteria should the nurse include when obtaining an older adult client's informed consent for a procedure?
Select all that apply:

[ ] 1. Must be able to understand the procedures and the risks

[ ] 2. Must be able to consent voluntarily

[ ] 3. Must be mentally competent

[ ] 4. Must be able to live independently

[ ] 5. Must be able to write

[ ] 6. Must be able to discuss the procedure with the client's significant other

17. Which of the following four older adult clients should the nurse permit to sign a consent form?
1. A 66-year-old client who has received pain medication
2. A 78-year-old client who has a legal guardian
3. A 55-year-old client who has resided in a long-term care facility for 10 years
4. An 80-year-old client who is experiencing occasional memory loss

18. The nurse is caring for a terminally ill older adult client who may die soon. When the client's condition changes and the client becomes mentally incompetent, the nurse should consult which of the following?
1. The client's spouse
2. The client's children
3. The physician
4. Durable Power of Attorney for Health Care

19. To prevent being sued for unlawful restraint, which of the following is a priority for the nurse caring for an older adult?
1. Contact the physician for appropriate orders and chart the reason for using restraints
2. Communicate the reason for applying restraints to the family
3. Tie the restraints so the client has maximum movement
4. Communicate with the client about why restraints are being used

20. The nurse calls a 77-year-old client's physician to report a change in the client's condition and to request orders for a pain medication. The physician is unable to take the call and a message is left with the office receptionist. The call is returned one hour later by the receptionist, who repeats a verbal order from the physician. Which of the following is the most appropriate intervention?

    1. Insist on speaking to the physician personally

    2. Accept the order from the receptionist and document it appropriately

    3. Refuse to accept the order from the receptionist and call back later

    4. Accept the order as it comes from the physician as interpreted by the receptionist

21. A 93-year-old client's health is declining rapidly. There is no advance directive or Durable Power of Attorney for Health Care. In this case, the nurse should

    1. provide minimal care to prolong life.

    2. consult the agency ethics committee.

    3. wait for physician's orders to provide care.

    4. provide all measures available for the care of the client.

22. An older adult has had an advance directive drawn up in the event there is no hope of recovery from a terminal illness. A distant relative is present and wants all possible medical treatment given to prolong life. The nurse should

    1. follow the advance directive no matter what the relative wants.

    2. follow the instructions of the relative.

    3. contact the physician for a change of orders.

    4. consult all of the client's family members to determine what care they want provided.

23. The nurse observes bruises and skin tears on the older adult client. The client does not make eye contact and appears fearful. Which of the following is the priority nursing action?

    1. Document the findings

    2. Ask the client about the bruises and skin tears

    3. Call the physician

    4. Ask family members what has happened

24. A 75-year-old female client is brought to the emergency department with a fractured hip. The emergency services personnel report she was found at the bottom of a flight of steps in the basement of her ex-husband's home. The client, who is undernourished (less than 10th percentile for weight),

tells the nurse that she lives in the basement and her ex-husband takes care of her and her finances. The nurse should

1. report the case to the elder abuse hotline for potential neglect and abuse.

2. wait for the physician to decide if a referral should be made.

3. make no report or referral because there is not enough evidence.

4. ask the client why she is so thin and lives in the basement.

25. An 84-year-old woman is brought to the emergency department by ambulance from a long-term care facility. The client has Stage III Alzheimer's-like dementia (ALD). She is rubbing her lower abdomen and moaning. A sterile urine specimen is obtained as part of the physical assessment. The laboratory technician calls the nurse with the results of the urinary analysis that are consistent with a urinary tract infection plus the presence of live sperm. The nurse should

1. call the long-term facility and ask what has happened to the client.

2. call the elder abuse hotline and follow the agency's rape protocol.

3. follow the instructions of the physician.

4. do what the nursing supervisor advises the nurse to do.

ANSWERS AND RATIONALES

1. 4. The registered nurse should immediately meet with the LPN and NA to stop the practice of the NA adjusting the intravenous infusion. Stopping a potentially dangerous practice is the priority. Informing the charge nurse and completing an occurrence report are the next actions.
   NP = Im
   CN = Sa/1
   CL = Ap
   SA = 8

2. 2. The nurse must act on information that the client is in danger. The nurse who does not further assess the client and make the appropriate referrals is negligent and liable. Negligence is the omission or commission of an act that departs from the acceptable and reasonable standards of practice. Malpractice is a type of negligence in which any unreasonable act or professional misconduct results in injury to the client. Beneficence is a principle that requires the nurse to act in ways that benefit the client. Nonmaleficence is similar to beneficence and requires the nurse to act in such a manner as to avoid causing harm to clients.
   NP = Ev
   CN = Sa/1
   CL = Ap
   SA = 8

3. 2. The nurse is expected to follow the standard of care at all times, which in this case is to follow universal precautions and agency policy. Negligence is the omission or commission of an act that departs from the acceptable and reasonable standards of practice. Malpractice is a type of negligence in which any unreasonable act or professional misconduct results in injury to the client. Coercion is an actual or implied threat of harm or penalty for not participating in a research project or receiving rewards for participating in a research project.

NP = An
CN = Sa/1
CL = Ap
SA = 8

4. 2. A client who would be appropriate to delegate to unlicensed assistive personnel is a client who had a cerebrovascular accident seven days ago. This would be an appropriate assignment because this client requires no specific care. A client with suspected pancreatitis and a blood sugar of 312 is unstable. A client who is in severe pain and has esophageal cancer requires prompt intervention, such as administration of an analgesic. A client who is dying also requires specific care, even though it is end-of-life care.

NP = Pl
CN = Sa/1
CL = An
SA = 8

5. 3. Clients have the right to give consent and the right to confidentiality. They should not be confined without consent, regardless of age. Emergency care is expected even if the client cannot give consent.

NP = Pl
CN = Sa/1
CL = An
SA = 8

6. standard of care. Standard of care is the degree of judgment and skill in nursing care that would be given by a reasonable and prudent professional nurse under similar circumstances. This is the same for clients of all ages.

NP = An
CN = Sa/1
CL = Ap
SA = 8

7. 1. The nurse must legally prescribe a medication for the purpose for which it was ordered. The nurse cannot prescribe the diphenhydramine (Benadryl) for restlessness within the scope of nursing practice. The nurse should further assess the client and contact the physician.

NP = Im
CN = Sa/1

CL = An
SA = 8

8. 3. The nurse's responsibility is to the client. The client's pain should be assessed and treated as prescribed, especially since the client has requested the medication. The daughter should discuss her concern with the health care team.
NP = Im
CN = Sa/1
CL = An
SA = 8

9. 3. The nurse in charge was responsible for the resident's safety. Even though the residents were "checked," the nurse should have provided for supervision.
NP = Ev
CN = Sa/1
CL = An
SA = 8

10. 2. The nurse should serve as a client advocate for the client in order to provide the client with the safest environment. The number 13 may cause the superstitious client to suffer emotional harm.
NP = Im
CN = Sa/1
CL = An
SA = 8

11. 3. The nurse had a responsibility to provide the physician with the information on the sulfa allergy reported by the client. The nurse should not have given the Septra. Negligence is the omission to do something that a reasonable person led by those ordinary considerations that ordinarily regulate human affairs would do or doing something another reasonable person would not do. Battery is unlawful touching of another person. Assault is an unjustifiable attempt or threat to touch a person without consent that results in fear of immediate harm. The touching may not actually occur. Malpractice is a type of negligence in which any unreasonable act or professional misconduct results in injury to the client.
NP = An
CN = Sa/1
CL = Ap
SA = 8

12. 2. Defamation of character is an oral or written communication to a third party that damages a person's reputation, such as stating when transferring a client, "He's a dirty old man. Watch out!"
NP = Im
CN = Sa/1

CL = Ap

SA = 8

13. 4. The nurse cannot take the client's property without the client's permission. The ginger could be part of the client's ethnicity and should be honored. Taking the ginger away from the client could be theft.

NP = Im

CN = Sa/1

CL = Ap

SA = 8

14. 3. The registered nurse should assess the newly unstable client. The assessment should be performed before notifying the physician. The UAP may be asked to stay with a client who is confused, but this is not the priority. An LPN should not be assigned to assess or care for a client whose condition is unstable and changing.

NP = Im

CN = Sa/1

CL = An

SA = 8

15. 3. A nurse who fails to turn an older adult client as ordered is violating the standards of practice. There are standards of practice to prevent skin breakdown mandating repositioning every two hours.

NP = Ev

CN = Sa/1

CL = Ap

SA = 8

16. 1,2,3. In order to give informed consent, the client must be able to understand the procedure and the risks, be able to consent voluntarily, and be mentally competent. The ability to live independently or to discuss the procedure with a significant other has no bearing on the ability to give informed consent for a procedure or surgery. The client does not have to be able to write. The client may be able to make an X.

NP = Pl

CN = Sa/1

CL = Ap

SA = 8

17. 3. A legal guardian precludes the client's ability to make decisions. The guardian must give permission for all aspects of the client's care. If a client has memory loss or confusion, then consent cannot be gained. A client who has received pain medication cannot sign a consent form. The fact that a client has been in a long-term care facility for 10 years does not alter the client's ability to sign the consent form.

NP = An
CN = Sa/1
CL = An
SA = 8

18. 4. When the client can no longer make personal health care decisions, guidance is given to the health care team, specifically the nurse who is caring for the dying client, by the Durable Power of Attorney for Health Care. This document names the individual specified by the client to make end-of-life care decisions.
NP = Im
CN = Sa/1
CL = Ap
SA = 8

19. 1. Communicating with the physician and obtaining appropriate orders for using restraints are essential. Following agency protocol and standards of care for the use of restraints is necessary. Communication with the client and family is crucial, but not the priority.
NP = Im
CN = Sa/1
CL = Ap
SA = 8

20. 1. When a receptionist calls an order back on behalf of the physician, the nurse should insist on talking to the physician. With that being said, agency personnel should direct the nurse on how to handle physician's orders that are relayed through a nonlicensed person, in this case a receptionist. In home care and long-term care, the nurse may find it a time-consuming action to actually find and speak to a physician directly.
NP = Im
CN = Sa/1
CL = Ap
SA = 8

21. 4. The fact that the client is 93 years old is insufficient reason to withhold care when there is no advance directive or Durable Power of Attorney for Health Care. Until the ethical and legal ramifications of prolonging this client's life have been legally determined, the nurse should provide all care possible. A "slow code" is neither ethical or legal.
NP = Im
CN = Sa/1
CL = Ap
SA = 8

22. 1. An advance directive is written instruction that states which health care treatments should be performed or withheld or that designates someone to act on the client's behalf if decision-making capacity becomes impaired. The nurse should advocate for the client's wishes. The relative can discuss the matter with the client and other family members.
NP = Im
CN = Sa/1
CL = Ap
SA = 8

23. 2. After discovering skin tears on an older adult client, it is a priority that the nurse gain more information from the client. Next, the nurse should assess the client for other injuries. It is mandatory that the nurse report suspected abuse and neglect to the state's elder abuse hotline. The older adult must be removed from a dangerous situation. Asking the family members about the injuries may cause further abuse if the family is the source of the abuse.
NP = Im
CN = Sa/1
CL = Ap
SA = 8

24. 1. The nurse is a mandatory reporter of suspected elder abuse or neglect. Because the client is undernourished and has sustained a serious injury, the nurse is warranted in making a report or referral to the elder abuse hotline. An investigation will be made. The nurse should not wait until another member of the health care team decides if a referral should be made.
NP = Im
CN = Sa/1
CL = Ap
SA = 8

25. 2. The nurse should carefully document the assessment of the client. The elder abuse hotline must be called in order to activate the system to protect the client from abuse or rape. A client with Stage III Alzheimer's-like dementia is not able to give consent for sexual intercourse and has been raped.
NP = Im
CN = Sa/1
CL = Ap
SA = 8